INFECTION CONTROL POLICIES AND PROCEDURES FOR COMMUNITY PSARAMEDICINE AND MIH *SECOND EDITION*

INFECTION CONTROL POLICIES AND PROCEDURES FOR COMMUNITY PARAMEDICINE AND MIH *SECOND EDITION*

KATHERINE H. WEST

FIRE ENGINEERING · BOOKS ·

Disclaimer
The recommendations, advice, descriptions, and methods in this book are presented solely for educational purposes. Photos are for instructional purposes only. Always wear the proper level of approved PPE when conducting training drills and operating at incidents. The author and publisher assume no liability whatsoever for any loss or damage that results from the use of any of the material in this book. Use of the material in this book is solely at the risk of the user.

Copyright © 2026 by
Fire Engineering Books
110 S. Hartford Ave., Suite 200
Tulsa, Oklahoma 74120 USA

800.752.9764
+1.918.831.9421
info@fireengineeringbooks.com
www.FireEngineeringBooks.com

Executive Vice President: Eric Schlett
Vice President, Group Publishing: Amanda Champion
Vice President of Content Operations: Starlet Franz
Sales and Customer Service Manager: Lane Nash
Managing Editors: Diane Rothschild and David Rhodes
Production Manager: Tony Quinn
Senior Development Editor: Daniel Edward Petrino
Book Designer: Robert Kern, TIPS Publishing Services, Carrboro, NC
Cover Designer: Brandon Ash

ISBN: 9781593705237

Library of Congress Cataloging-in-Publication Data Available on Request

All rights reserved. No part of this book may be reproduced, stored in a retrieval system, or transcribed in any form or by any means, electronic or mechanical, including photocopying and recording, without the prior written permission of the publisher.

Printed in the United States of America

1 2 3 4 5   30 29 28 27 26

To Jim

Thank you for all your support and assistance

Contents

Acknowledgments ix
Introduction xi

1. **Regulatory Aspects for Community Paramedicine and Mobile-Integrated Health Care** 1
   Understanding Government Rules and Regulations Applicable to Fire and Emergency Medical Services 1

2. **Basic Infection Control Practices for Emergency Medical Service Providers and Patients** 5
   Vaccines and Immunizations 5
   Protecting Patients, Coworkers, and Yourself 7
   Work Restriction Guidelines 8
   Work Restrictions for COVID-19 13

3. **Basic Personal Protective Measures for Use in Home Care** 15
   The Hierarchy of Safety Controls 15
   Handwashing 16

4. **Exposure Issues in the Community Paramedicine and Mobile-Integrated Health Work Setting** 21
   Defining Exposures 21
   Post-Exposure Procedures in Home Care 22
   Scope of Practice 22
   Bloodborne Exposures 23
   Airborne and Droplet Exposures 25

5. **Basic Personal Protective Equipment in Home Care**........ 27
   Transmission-Based Precautions..29
   Cleaning Patient Care Equipment......................................31

6. **Patient Care Infection Control and General Health**......... 33
   Caring for Patients with Multidrug-Resistant Infections................38
   Assessment for Diabetic Foot Ulcers 46
   General Cleaning 49
   Razors and Fingerstick Pens 49
   Wound Irrigation 51
   Specimen Transport to Lab 52
   Disposal of Discontinued Medications 52
   Assessment of Patient Infection.......................................52
   Definitions of Infection in Home Care Setting.........................54
   Reporting Patient Infection 60
   Administration of Vaccines and Immunizations..........................61
   Compliance Monitoring...68

Index 77

Acknowledgments

Thank you for your time, Michael R. Wilcox, MD, FACEP, FAAFP. Dr. Wilcox serves as the Medical Director for EMS Programs at Hennepin Technical College and South Central Technical College and as the Medical Advisor of EMS Programs for the Minnesota State College and University System.

Thank you to the CDC Clinicians PEP Hotline for their assistance in the development of post-exposure medical follow-up and testing issues for this developing care environment.

Introduction

The Affordable Care Act has opened the door for emergency medical services (EMS) to expand the delivery of services to underserved rural communities. The Center for Medicare and Medicaid Services (CMS) is now reducing medical facility reimbursement by 3% for frequent readmissions. The rate has increased since 2015 and amounts to a significant sum of money.

CMS is also not reimbursing medical facilities for healthcare-associated infections (HAIs). HAIs are those which occur two days after hospital admission and are unrelated to the patient's admitting diagnosis. Medical facilities will also not be reimbursed for infections that occur up to 30 days after discharge. Since nonreimbursement began in 2009, hospital infection rates have been on the decline. That was until the COVID-19 pandemic, which started in 2019. HAIs increased as focus turned solely to dealing with the pandemic. Now, facilities are working to return to prepandemic practices.[1]

Recent studies have revealed that patients are being discharged without receiving or fully understanding their discharge instructions. This single omission can lead to the patient needing to be readmitted. CMS will now require that the patient's medical chart contain a copy of their discharge instructions. These will be important references for in-home care providers.

How do each of these issues impact the provision of EMS services? First, having effective infection control practices, up-to-date vaccines and immunizations, proper cleaning and disinfection of equipment, and suitable work restriction guidelines in place for EMS providers is a start. With the basics in place, departments can then move on to expanding services to the community.

Second, departments that are looking to expand services to meet the needs of the elderly, disabled, and those living in rural areas where health care is not easily accessible will need to refocus and expand infection control practices applicable to the home care environment. This may require changes in scope of practice.

Third, medical facilities are looking toward EMS as the possible source for patient infections. Documentation and compliance-monitoring programs will serve as liability reduction and risk management tools.

Fourth, EMS is now under the scope of healthcare-associated infections. The new term, HAI, is much broader and applies to more healthcare delivery services.

The cost of an HAI is significant. Here are a few examples:[2]

- C. diff: $11,285 per patient
- Central line infection: $45,814 per patient
- Wound infection: $20,785 per patient
- Ventilator-associated pneumonia: $40,144 per patient
- Catheter-associated urinary tract infection: $603–$1,189 per patient

A recent study published in the *American Journal of Infection Control* reported a final analysis of 199,462 patients from 8,255 home health agencies. The study revealed that approximately 3.5% of patients developed infections while in home health care. These infections lead to the need for emergency care or hospitalization. Infections in home healthcare patients varied by agencies, and these variances may have been due to differences in infection control practices and the use of an infection surveillance system.

The focus of this publication is to address infection control issues in the mobile health unit and community paramedicine work setting to prevent hospital readmissions and promote quality care for the patients that are served.

Objectives

1. Identify key infection control measures for EMS protection.
2. Identify key infection control measures for patient protection in the home care environment.
3. Review transmission-based precautions.
4. Cite proper procedure for exposure reporting for community paramedicine and mobile-integrated health care.
5. Review listing or reportable diseases.
6. Identify signs of infection in home care.
7. Review medical waste regulations for home care.
8. Develop a system for tracking readmissions.
9. Develop a system for tracking postdischarge infections.
10. Develop a system for disposal of unused medications.
11. Developing a procedure for postexposure source patient testing in the home care environment.

Notes

1. "CMS Proposes Rule to Improve Health Equity and Care Quality in Hospitals," Centers for Medicare and Medicaid Services, June 13, 2016, https://www.cms.gov/newsroom/press-releases/cms-proposes-rule-improve-health-equity-and-care-quality-hospitals.
2. Eyal Zimlichman et al. "Health Care-Associated Infections: A Meta-analysis of Cost and Financial Impact on the U.S. Health-Care System," *JAMA Intern Med 173*, vol. 22 (2013): 2039–2046. https://doi.org/10.1001/jamainternmed.2013.9763.

Regulatory Aspects for Community Paramedicine and Mobile-Integrated Health Care

Understanding Government Rules and Regulations Applicable to Fire and Emergency Medical Services

The Ryan White Law

There are several government rules and regulations that apply to community paramedicine (CP) and mobile-integrated health care just as they apply to traditional fire and emergency medical services. Perhaps one of the most important was the passage of the Ryan White Comprehensive AIDS Resources Emergency Act by the U.S. Congress in 1990. The focus of this piece of legislation was funding for human immunodeficiency virus (HIV) or acquired immunodeficiency syndrome (known as AIDS) services. However, a section was added to this bill which applies to emergency response employers. This newly added section requires that every employer of an emergency response agency appoint a "designated officer." This position is more commonly known as the *designated infection control officer* (DICO). This individual is responsible for managing exposure events involving department employees.

Designated officers serve to ensure that an exposed employee receives proper care and counseling following an exposure event. Many administrative personnel do not realize that whomever the department chooses to render care for postexposure medical treatment only acts as an agent on behalf of the department, and the department holds liability if proper care and counseling are not rendered to the exposed employee. This holds true in the case of any exposure, be it airborne, droplet-transmitted, or bloodborne, in both CP and mobile-integrated healthcare situations.

The Ryan White Law lists the bloodborne, airborne, and droplet-transmitted diseases that medical facilities are required to conduct source patient testing for if the medical facility suspects or diagnoses a disease on the list. The disease list was updated in 2011, and will be presented in a subsequent chapter of this book. It should also be noted that in the 2011 updated list, a new category was added for clarification—droplet-transmitted diseases. That is very important as diseases such as COVID-19 and N. Meningitis were added. This clarification has been essential in identifying how diseases are transmitted.

The designated officer is tasked with making the first call as to whether an incident meets the criteria for an exposure. The DICO then works with the emergency department to obtain source patient testing. The Ryan White Law primarily deals with patients who are transported. However, in both CP and mobile-integrated healthcare environments, the DICO would contact the patient's attending physician to obtain orders for source patient testing. This means that the process must be adjusted to meet the needs of this new care environment. A detailed process for postexposure follow-up will be presented in detail in the postexposure chapter in this book.[1]

The Occupational Safety and Health Administration

The Occupational Safety and Health Act of 1970 created the department of Occupational Safety and Health (OSHA). OSHA is the governing body responsible for ensuring safe and healthy working conditions in the United States. Of most importance is the General Duty Clause—Section 5(a). This clause states,

> Each employer shall furnish to each of his employees' employment and a place of employment which are free from recognized hazards that are causing or are likely to cause death or serious physical harm to his employees.

OSHA has legal authority over federal government employers as of an executive order issued in 1980. State and local governments are not directly under OSHA, but most state governments have passed legislation requiring OSHA compliance.

The General Duty Clause also includes Section 5(b), addressing the responsibilities of employees. This section states,

> Each employee shall comply with occupational safety and health standards and all rules, regulations, and orders issued pursuant to this Act which are applicable to his own actions and conduct.

This shows that employees share a role in their own safety.

Both Section 5(a) and Section 5(b) are applicable to all employers of healthcare providers. OSHA and the Centers for Disease Control and Prevention (CDC) list emergency medical service personnel in the definition of healthcare personnel.

The General Duty Clause gives OSHA the legal authority to issue citations and fines for workplace hazards that are not covered by existing OSHA regulations. For example, OSHA is using the General Duty Clause to enforce many of the CDC guidelines.

CDC guidelines that are currently being enforced by OSHA include guidelines on tuberculosis, work restriction, vaccines and immunizations, and post-exposure medical follow-up.

Medical facilities fall under federal OSHA jurisdiction, as they are private entities. Fire and emergency medical services usually fall under state and local government. More than half of the states cover public safety personnel under OSHA. There are some states that have passed legislation covering state and local government employees who might not otherwise have OSHA protection.

The General Duty Clause also has a Part B. This section addresses employee responsibilities regarding compliance. This section states, "Each employee shall comply with occupational safety and health standards and all rules, regulations, and orders issued pursuant to this Act which are applicable to his own actions and conduct." This is the reference for conducting compliance monitoring. Compliance monitoring is to be part of the Exposure Control Plan.[2] It is important to be aware of OSHA jurisdiction in your state.

State HIV Testing Laws

Each state has an HIV testing law. Some states require patient consent to test for HIV, and others have an exception to consent if there has been a healthcare worker exposure. There are several states such as Kansas, Maine, Massachusetts, New Hampshire, New Mexico, Oregon, and Washington which require obtaining a court order to test for HIV if the patient does not consent. HIV is the only disease that raises consent issues. There is no consent issue for testing for hepatitis B, hepatitis C, or syphilis.[3]

State Medical Waste Regulations

Each state has their own medical waste regulations. These are specific with regard to defining what is considered medical waste and how it should be handled for disposal. OSHA is to follow the state's regulations. Sharps are always considered to be medical waste, however there are exceptions in how they are disposed of in the home care setting. Gloves, for the most part, are not considered to be medical waste. This illustrates the importance of knowing the definitions in your specific state.[4] Following the definition in your state will lower costs associated with disposal of medical waste.

Notes

1. Ryan White Comprehensive AIDS Resources Emergency (CARE) Act, Pub. L. No. 101–308, 104 Stat. 576 (1990).
2. Occupational Safety and Health Act of 1970, 29 U.S.C. § 654.
3. "State Laws That Address High-Impact HIV Prevention Efforts," March 17, 2022, Centers for Disease Control & Prevention.
4. Enforcement Procedures for the Occupational Exposure to Bloodborne Pathogens. CPL 02-02-069. Occupational Safety and Health Administration, 2001. https://www.osha.gov/sites/default/files/enforcement/directives/CPL_02-02-069.pdf

Basic Infection Control Practices for Emergency Medical Service Providers and Patients

Vaccines and Immunizations

Basic infection control for care providers begins with personal and patient protection. This involves participation in recommended vaccine and immunization practices for healthcare personnel.

It is important to note that both the Centers for Disease Control and Prevention (CDC) and the Occupational Safety and Health Administration (OSHA) clearly list emergency medical service (EMS) personnel as healthcare personnel.[1]

Many EMS providers need boosters or revaccination for some diseases. For example, all healthcare personnel are required to have received a one-time booster for tetanus, diphtheria, and acellular pertussis (Tdap). Pertussis (whooping cough) is back in large numbers across the country. EMS personnel should not pose a risk to coworkers or patients in the community that are being served, therefore, receiving the Tdap booster is important. Employers are required to offer and pay for preventative vaccines. Employers cannot require employees to use their own health insurance to cover costs unless the employer pays the full insurance premium and any copays.[2]

Persons who were vaccinated against measles, mumps, and rubella (MMR) between 1963–1967 need to be revaccinated. The vaccine administered during this time was a killed-virus vaccine, which have been shown not to be protective. EMS personnel in this group need to be vaccinated with two doses of the live measles vaccine, given one month apart. EMS personnel who have documentation of having MMR are protected by acquired immunity. Those who were vaccinated are also protected for life.[3]

Current vaccine, immunization, and testing requirements for EMS personnel include the following:

- Hepatitis B vaccine
- tuberculosis (TB) testing
- MMR vaccine

- Chickenpox vaccine
- Tdap booster
- Seasonal flu vaccine
- COVID-19 vaccine (as of 2020)

Each vaccine is to be offered to employees who are not protected. Current department members are to be asked to give their vaccine and childhood disease status for their medical record. New hires are provided this information during the hiring process. Those who are not protected are to be offered protective vaccines. Employees have the right to decline vaccines but must sign a declination form. This is to document that the employer met their responsibility to offer the vaccine. Remember—signing a declination form is important for the employer.

TB testing has changed a great deal over the past few years. TB testing is to be performed on hire and not again unless an exposure occurs.[4] TB testing frequency began to change starting in 2005, and in May of 2019, the CDC published their latest guidance.[5] OSHA enforces the CDC tuberculosis guidelines using the General Duty Clause.

The newest and most accurate form of TB testing is the blood test. This has been available since 2004, and it was then that the CDC recommended this as the method for screening healthcare personnel, including fire and EMS. Currently there are two TB blood tests available in the marketplace: QuantiFERON-TB and T-Spot TB. Since TB testing is to be performed at the time of hiring, new employees have blood drawn as part of their physical exam for hire. More blood is then drawn and sent to the laboratory for analysis. Accurate results are available in 24 hours.

Each department must offer and pay for these vaccines. Vaccines are to be administered at no cost to the employee.

An employer cannot require an employee to use their own health insurance to pay for any needed vaccines. This means that unless an employer pays for an employee's full insurance coverage and any copay costs, the employer must pay. This is stated in the OSHA Compliance Directive document, CPL 02-02-069.[6] If an individual does not wish to receive protective vaccines, a declination form must be signed.

Declination forms do not remove employee rights. They are documentation that the department has met its requirement to offer vaccines to those who are not protected. The need for declination forms is also addressed in National Fire Protection Association (NFPA) 1581 Standard and the CDC vaccination guidelines.

It is important to be aware that many CDC Guidelines are enforced by OSHA. This is accomplished using the General Duty Clause of the OSH Act of 1970 under Section 5, Duties Part A.

The goal of vaccine programs is to offer protection from diseases for which there is a preventative vaccine.

EMS training programs requiring vaccinations prior to entry will be very helpful for departments, This will result in new hires coming to departments already vaccinated. which will lower department costs.

Medical facilities have stated that EMS personnel who have signed declination forms for recommended vaccines will not be permitted to take part in clinical rotations.

Vaccine records are to be part of the employee's medical record and be able to be accessed by the DICO 24/7.[7] This is to establish the employee's status if an exposure occurs and direct the start of postexposure medical follow-up.

For example, if there is an exposure to a hepatitis B positive patient, it is crucial to know if the employee has received the hepatitis B vaccine. With that information, the DICO will know which of the five postexposure protocols should be used for postexposure follow-up.[8]

> If protected by vaccine, there is no concern if an exposure occurs.

Protecting Patients, Coworkers, and Yourself

Work restriction guidelines were first published by the CDC in 1999. In 2011, key provisions to these guidelines were updated before they were updated again in 2020 to address COVID-19. The following is a combination of the two documents, so there is a full list of the restrictions. NFPA 1581 refers to these CDC guidelines and they are being enforced by OSHA using the General Duty Clause of the OSH Act of 1970.[9]

As you'll remember from chapter 1, the General Duty Clause Section 5(a) states that,

> Employers are required to provide their employees with a place of employment that is free from recognizable hazards that are causing or likely to cause death or serious harm to employees.

The Society for Human Resource Management stated in 2013 that employees who come to work while ill pose a direct threat to others and thus the General Duty Clause applies.

Studies have revealed that healthcare workers in almost all disciplines are aware that coming to work when ill puts others at risk, but they continue to work when ill.

Section 5(b) of the General Duty Clause states that,

> Each employee shall comply with occupational safety and health standards and all rules, regulations, and orders issued pursuant to this Act which are applicable to his own actions and conduct.

Thus, employees clearly share a role in following work restriction guidelines.

A new issue that has arisen in work restrictions is tattoos. A new tattoo is an open area on the skin and needs to be covered until healed. Healing takes an average of 7 to 14 days. Healing time can be further lengthened by the tattoo's size and location. If the tattoo is too large to cover with dressing, then work restriction would be appropriate. Although tattoos are not specifically addressed in the work restriction guidelines, working with nonintact skin is addressed by OSHA, the CDC, and NFPA 1581.[10]

Work restriction guidelines are focused on patient care and might appear only to address the hospital setting, but they also apply to the EMS setting—especially to those working in community paramedicine and mobile-integrated healthcare settings. This can be found in the document "Immunization of Healthcare Personnel in the definition of healthcare care personnel."[11] EMS is listed on page 2 of this document.

Work Restriction Guidelines

Table 2–1 shows a summary of suggested work restrictions for healthcare personnel exposed to or infected with infectious diseases of importance in healthcare settings, in the absence of state and local regulations (modified from Advisory Committee on Immunization Practices [ACIP] recommendations).[12]

Table 2–1. CDC Personnel Health Guidelines: Suggested work restrictions for healthcare personnel exposed to or infected with infectious diseases of importance in healthcare settings, in the absence of state and local regulations (modified from ACIP recommendations; combination of 1997, 2011, and 2022 versions).[13]

Disease or Problem	Work restriction	Duration
Conjunctivitis	Restrict from patient contact and contact with the patient's environment	Until discharge ceases
COVID-19 Virus	In most higher risk exposures, no work restriction regardless of vaccination status	10 days if the exposed person cannot be tested, wear source control, or is immunocompromised

Disease or Problem	Work restriction	Duration
Cytomegalovirus infections	No restriction	
Diarrheal diseases		
Acute stage (diarrhea with other symptoms)	Restrict from patient contact, contact with the patient's environment, or food handling	Until symptoms resolve
Convalescent stage, *Salmonella* spp.	Restrict from care of high-risk patients	Until symptoms resolve; consult with local patents and state health authorities regarding need for negative stool cultures
Diphtheria	Exclude from duty	Until antimicrobial therapy completed, and 2 cultures obtained[3] 24 hours apart are negative
Ebola Virus (and other hemorrhagic fevers)	Determine whether physical exposure actually occurred Follow CDC guidelines Monitor to assess the presence of fever or other symptomatology	Through day 21 post exposure
Enteroviral infections	Restrict from care of infants, neonates, and immunocompromised patients and their environments	Until symptoms resolve
Hepatitis A	Restrict from patient contact, contact with patient's environment, and food handling	Until 7 days after onset of jaundice
Hepatitis B		
Personnel with acute or chronic hepatitis B surface antigenemia who do not perform exposure-prone procedures	No restrictions[a]; refer to state regulations; standard precautions should always be observed	
Personnel with acute or chronic hepatitis B an antigenemia who perform exposure-prone procedures	Do not perform expsure-prone invasive procedures until counsel from an expert review panel has been sought; panel should review and recommend procedures the worker can perform, taking into account specific procedure as well as still and technique of worker; refer to state regulations	Until hepatitis B antigen is negative
Hepatitis C	No recommendation	

(continues)

Table 2–1. (*Continued*)

Disease or Problem	Work restriction	Duration
Herpes simplex		
Genital	No restriction	
Hands (herpetic window)	Restrict from patient contact and contact with the patient's environment	Until lesions heal
Orofacial	Evaluate need to restrict from care of high-risk patients	
Human immunodeficiency virus	Do not perform exposure-prone invasive procedures until counsel from an expert review panel has been sought; panel should review and recommend procedures the worker can perform; taking into account specific procedure as well as skill and technique of worker; standard precautions should always be observed; refer to state regulations	
Measles		
Active	Exclude from duty	Until 4 days after the rash appears
Post exposure (susceptible personnel)	Exclude from duty	From 5th day after 1st exposure through 21st day after last exposure or 4 days after rash appears
Meningococcal infections	Exclude from duty	Until 24 hours after start of effective therapy
Mumps		
Active	Exclude from duty	Until 5 days after onset of parotitis
Post exposure (susceptible personnel)	Exclude from duty	10 days after first exposure through 25 days after last exposure or 5 days after onset of parotitis
Pediculosis	Restrict from patient contact	Until treated and observed to be free of adult and immature lice
Pertussis[b]		
Active	Exclude from duty	Beginning of catarrhal stage through third week after onset of paroxysms or until 5 days after start of effective antimicrobial therapy
Post exposure (asymptomatic personnel)	Protection may have waned	Postexposure treatment may be helpful

Disease or Problem	Work restriction	Duration
Post exposure (symptomatic personnel)	Exclude from duty	5 days after start of effective antimicrobial therapy
Symptomatic personnel	Exclude from duty	
Asymptomatic healthcare professional (HCP) likely to expose a patient at risk for severe pertussis	No restriction from duty; on antimicrobial prophylactic therapy	
Asymptomatic personnel—other HCP	No restriction from duty; can receive postexposure prophylaxis or be monitored for 21 days after pertussis exposure and treated at the onset of signs and symptoms of pertussis	
Rubella		
Active	Exclude from duty	
Post exposure (personnel without evidence of rubella immunity)	Exclude from duty unless receipt of the second dose within 3–5 days after exposure	7 days after first exposure through 23 days after last exposure or 7 days after rash appears
Scabies		
Active	Exclude from duty	Until 24 hours after application of effective treatment
***Staphylococcus aureus* infection**	Exclude from duty	Until medically cleared
Active, draining skin lesions	Restrict from contact with patients and patient's environment of food handling	Until lesions have resolved
Carrier state	No restriction, unless personnel are epidemiologically linked to transmission of the organism	
Streptococcal infection, group A	Restrict from patient care, contact with patient's environment, or food handling	Until 24 hours after adequate treatment started
Tuberculosis		
Active disease	Exclude from duty	Until proved noninfectious
Purified-protein derivative converter	No restriction	
Varicella[c]		
Active	Exclude from duty	Until all lesions dry and crust; if only lesions that do not crust (i.e., macules and papules), until no new lesions appear within a 24-hour period

(continues)

Table 2–1. (Continued)

Disease or Problem	Work restriction	Duration
Post exposure (susceptible personnel)	Exclude from duty	8th day after 1st exposure through 21st day (28th day if varicella-zoster immune globulin administered) after the last exposure; if varicella occurs, until all lesions dry and crust or, if only lesions that do not crust (i.e., macules and papules), until no new lesions appear within a 24-hour period
Herpes Zoster		
Localized, in healthy person	Cover lesions; restrict from care of high-risk patients[d]	Until all lesions dry and crust
Generalized or localized in immunosuppressed person.	Exclude from duty	Until dissemination is ruled out
Post exposure (susceptible personnel)	Restrict from patient contact	From 10th day after 1st exposure through 21st day (28th day if VZIG given) after last exposure or, if varicella occurs, until all lesions dry and crust
Viral respiratory infections, acute febrile	Exclude from duty	Until afebrile ≥24 hours (without the use of fever-reducing medicines such as acetaminophen).[e,f]
HCP in contact with persons at high risk for complications of influenza		

[a]Persons who provide health care to patients or work in institutions that provide patient care (e.g., physicians, nurses, emergency medical personnel, dental professionals and students, medical and nursing students, laboratory technicians, hospital volunteers, and administrative and support staff in healthcare institutions).[14]

[b]Includes hospitalized neonates and pregnant women.

[c]Includes patients who are susceptible to varicella and at increased risk for complications of varicella (i.e., neonates, pregnant women, and immunocompromised persons of any age).

[d]Includes children aged <5 years, adults aged ≥65 years, pregnant women, American Indians and Alaska Natives, persons aged <19 years who are receiving long-term aspirin therapy, and persons with certain high-risk medical conditions (i.e., asthma, neurologic and neurodevelopmental conditions, chronic lung disease, heart disease, blood disorders, endocrine disorders, kidney disorders, liver disorders, metabolic disorders, weakened immune system due to disease or medication, and morbid obesity).

[e]Those with ongoing respiratory symptoms should be considered for evaluation by occupational health to determine appropriateness of contact with patients. If returning to care for patients in a protective environment (e.g., hematopoietic stem cell transplant patients), consider for temporary reassignment or exclusion from work for 7 days from symptom onset or until the resolution of symptoms, whichever is longer.

[f]Those who develop acute respiratory symptoms without fever should be considered for evaluation by occupational health to determine appropriateness of contact with patients and can be allowed to work unless caring for patients in a protective environment; these personnel should be considered for temporary reassignment or exclusion from work for 7 days from symptom onset or until the resolution of all non-cough symptoms, whichever is longer. If symptoms such as cough and sneezing are still present, HCP should wear a facemask during patient care activities. The importance of performing frequent hand hygiene (especially before and after each patient contact) should be reinforced.

Work Restrictions for COVID-19

In most circumstances, asymptomatic healthcare professionals (HCPs) with higher-risk exposures do not require work restriction. *Higher-risk exposures generally involve exposure of HCP's eyes, nose, or mouth to material potentially containing SARS-CoV-2, particularly if these HCP were present in the room for an aerosol-generating procedure.* Work restriction is not necessary for most asymptomatic HCPs following a higher-risk exposure, regardless of vaccination status.

Examples of when work restriction may be considered include the following:

- HCP is unable to be tested or wear source control as recommended for the 10 days following their exposure.
- HCP is moderately to severely immunocompromised.
- HCP cares for or works on a unit with patients who are moderately to severely immunocompromised.
- HCP works on a unit experiencing ongoing SARS-CoV-2 transmission that is not controlled with initial interventions.

If work restriction is recommended, HCP could return to work after either of the following time periods:

- HCP can return to work after 7 days following the exposure (day 0) if they do not develop symptoms and all viral testing as described for asymptomatic HCP following a higher-risk exposure is negative.
- If viral testing is not performed, HCP can return to work 10 days following the exposure if they do not develop symptoms.

In May 2024, the CDC stated that these guidelines for COVID-19 remain unchanged.

> In the provision of health care, we have a responsibility to protect the patients we serve in our communities as well as coworkers and ourselves.

Notes

1. "Immunization of Health Care Personnel," November, 2011, Centers for Disease Control & Prevention.
2. "Updated Recommendations for TB Screening, Testing, and Treatment of U.S. Health Care Personnel." May, 2019, Centers for Disease Control & Prevention.

3. "Updated Recommendations for TB Screening, Testing, and Treatment of U.S. Health Care Personnel."
4. "Updated Recommendations for TB Screening, Testing, and Treatment of U.S. Health Care Personnel."
5. Enforcement Procedures for the Occupational Exposure to Bloodborne Pathogens. CPL 02-02-069. Occupational Safety and Health Administration, 2001. https://www.osha.gov/sites/default/files/enforcement/directives/CPL_02-02-069.pdf.
6. Enforcement Procedures for the Occupational Exposure to Bloodborne Pathogens.
7. "Immunization of Health Care Personnel."
8. Sarah Schillie, Claudia Vellozzi, Arthur Reingold, et al., "Prevention of Hepatitis B Virus Infection in the United States: Recommendations of the Advisory Committee on Immunization Practices," *Morbidity and Mortality Weekly Report Recommendations and Reports* 67, no. 1 (2018): 1–31, http://doi.org/10.15585/mmwr.rr6701a1.
9. *NFPA 1581: Standard on Fire Department Infection Control Program,* Fire Engineering Books (2022).
10. *NFPA 1581: Standard on Fire Department Infection Control Program.*
11. "Immunization of Health-Care Personnel"; "Recommendations of the Advisory Committee on Immunization practices (APIC)," Morbidity and Mortality Weekly Report, November 25, 2011.
12. "Infection Control in Healthcare Personnel: Epidemiology and Control of Selected Infections Transmitted Among Healthcare Personnel and Patients," January 31, 2025, Centers for Disease Control & Prevention.
13. "Recommendations for Preventing Transmission of Human Immunodeficiency Virus and Hepatitis B Virus to Patients During Exposure-Prone Invasive Procedures," *Morbidity and Mortality Weekly Report Recommendations and Reports* 40, no. 8 (1991); Julia Garner et al., *Guideline for Isolation Precautions in Hospitals and CDC Guideline for Infection Control in Hospital Personnel* (Centers for Disease Control, 1983); "Immunization of Health-Care Workers: Recommendations of the Advisory Committee on Immunization Practices (ACIP) and the Hospital Infection Control Practices Advisory Committee (HICPAC)," *Morbidity and Mortality Weekly Report Recommendations and Reports* 46, no. 18 (1997).
14. "Immunization of Health-Care Workers"

Basic Personal Protective Measures for Use in Home Care

The Hierarchy of Safety Controls

The Hierarchy of Controls (figure 3–1) is used by the Centers for Disease Control (CDC) and the Occupational Safety and Health Administration to illustrate that personal protective equipment (PPE) can be effective barriers to transmission of infections but are secondary to the more effective measures such as administrative and engineering controls.

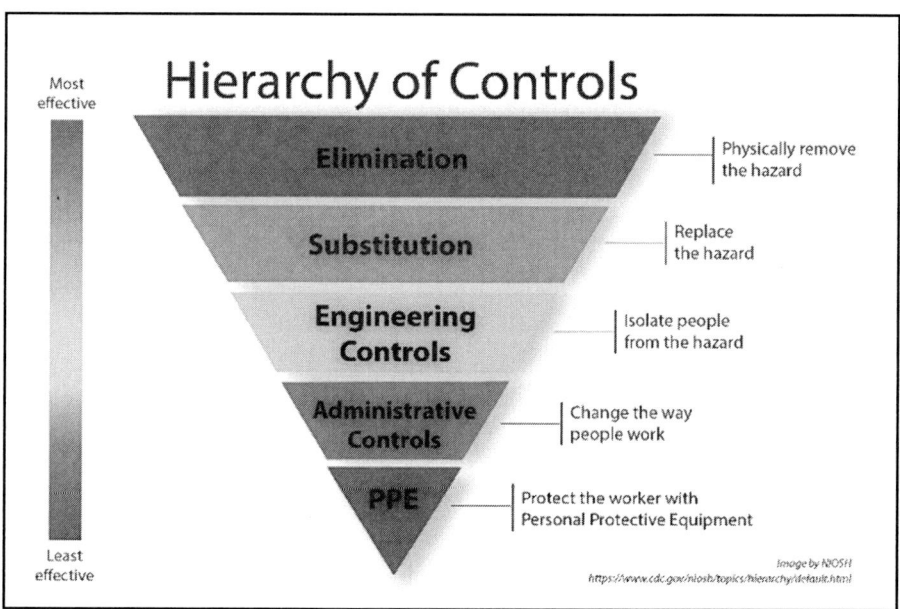

Figure 3–1. The Hierarchy of Controls used by the CDC and Occupational Safety and Health Administration (courtesy of Occupational Safety and Health Academy)

First, safety begins with the goal of eliminating risk. However, eliminating all exposure does not seem realistic in health care. The focus will be on minimizing risk for exposure and disease transmission. Many practices differ in the provision of home care. This can be explained and illustrated by a review of the safety pyramid.

The second level of safety is engineering controls. An example would be the requirement for the use of needle safe devices. Congress passed the Needlestick Safety and Prevention Law in 2000. Contaminated sharps injuries represented 80% of healthcare worker exposures. An example of an engineering control for protection from airborne and droplet disease is the use of the rear exhaust fan in the back of the ambulance. In the home care arena, opening windows would offer an example.

The third level addresses administrative controls. These would include vaccines and immunizations, education and training, the exposure control plan, and standard operating procedures.

The fourth and final level of the pyramid addresses the use of PPE.

The policies and procedures in the book are designed to address education and training and the development of standard operating procedures for use in the home care environment. Standard operating procedures for use in home care are similar to many used in the provision of emergency care but many are very different.

In December 2022, the CDC published a document titled "Core Infection & Control Practices for Safe Delivery of Healthcare in All Settings."[1] This document states, "PPE can be effective barriers to transmission of infections but are secondary to the more effective measures such as administrative and engineering controls."

Handwashing

Handwashing has long been established as the best measure for protection for both care providers and patients. However, study after study shows that healthcare workers do not comply with basic handwashing procedures. In two handwash studies involving emergency medical services personnel, this also appeared to be the case.

The first study was done in Texas and published in *Prehospital Emergency Care*.[2] The study was observational and was conducted by Dr. Bryan Bledsoe and colleagues. A total of 423 observations were conducted. The study noted that proper handwashing occurred in 27.8% of the observations.

Another study conducted at the Robert Woods Johnson University Hospital showed that there was 13% compliance with handwash practices.[3] This study

3 Basic Personal Protective Measures for Use in Home Care

was a survey of 1,500 emergency medical services providers. Remember that a survey involves self-reporting which could have influenced the results due to personal biases.

Both studies reflect handwash practices in emergency care. Would it be the same for in-home care? Let's work to ensure that proper handwashing is conducted (figure 3–2) and prevent infection in the patient that might result in hospital readmission (table 3–1).

> Handwashing remains your key prevention measure.

Four recently published studies show that when the use of gloves is decreased, compliance with handwashing increases. Overreliance on gloves has been a factor in the development of glove sensitivity and allergies.

This has been clearly established with latex, and now new allergy issues are related to the use of nitrile gloves.

Healthcare providers are reacting to some of the accelerators and color dyes that are used in nitrile gloves.

Note that gloves are not required or recommended for taking vital signs or giving an injection.

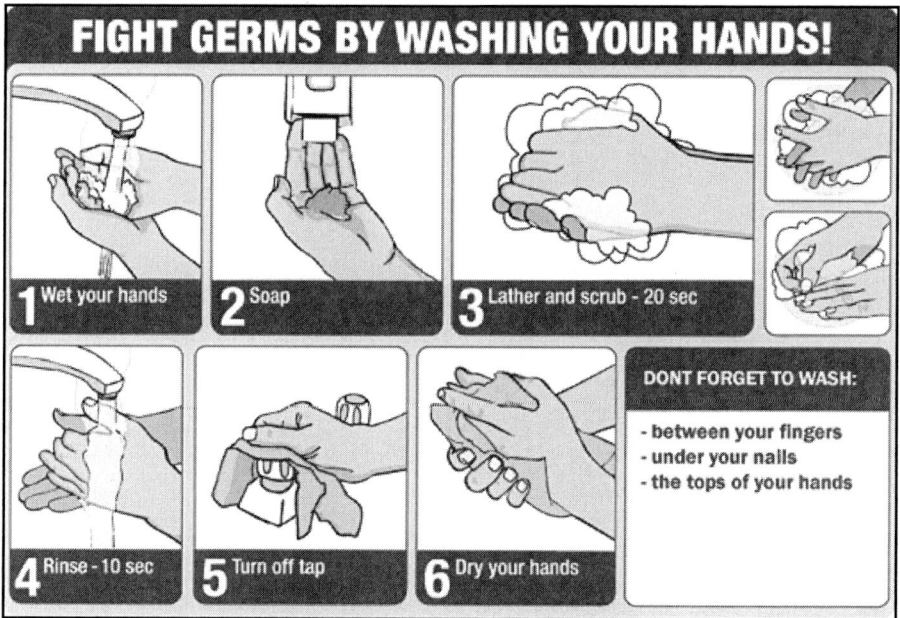

Figure 3–2. Proper handwashing procedure

Table 3–1. General and patient-specific handwashing care

Handwashing—General Care[a]	
Procedure	**Rationale and Action**
No artificial fingernails or extensions may be worn by direct patient care providers.	Artificial fingernails are linked to bacteria and fungi passed from care providers to patients.
No gel nails should be permitted.	Gel interferes with good hand washing technique.[b]
Hands must be washed before and after patient contact.	Handwashing is the single most important means of preventing the spread of infection.
Scrub hands for at least 15 seconds; use friction rub action after the soap is applied.	Friction will assist in the removal of dirt as well as bacteria and other organisms.
When running water is not available, use a waterless handwash solution.	Waterless alcohol-based agents such as: Alcare, Purell, Hibistat and Cal-Stat may be used.
Check active ingredient handwash solutions.	**No product containing Triclosan should be used because the FDA has pulled these products.**
Rinse hands well under running water.	**The routine use of antibacterial soap is NOT recommended.**
Dry with a paper towel.	
Use paper towel to turn off water faucet.	Faucets are handled by soiled hands.
Handwashing–C. diff Patient	
Handwashing is to be performed with warm water and plain soap.	C. diff is a spore forming agent and requires a chlorine-based product to kill the spore.
Handwashing–Norovirus Patient	
Handwashing is to be performed with water and plain soap.	Norovirus is a nonenveloped virus which is less susceptible to normal disinfection. Alcohol-based products do not kill norovirus.
Handwashing–Patient with Candia auris (C. auris)	
When caring for patients with C. auris, healthcare personnel should follow standard hand hygiene practices.	
Alcohol-based hand sanitizer is the preferred hand hygiene method for C. auris.	Use when hands are not visibly soiled. If hands are visibly soiled, wash with soap and water.

[a] "Guidelines for Hand Hygiene in Health Care Settings: Recommendations of the Healthcare Infection Control Practices Advisory Committee and the HICPAC/SHEA/APIC/IDSA Hand Hygiene Task Force," *Morbidity and Mortality Weekly Report* 51, RR16 (2002): 1–44, https://www.cdc.gov/mmwr/preview/mmwrhtml/rr5116a1.htm
[b] Angela Hewlett et al., "Evaluation of the bacterial burden of gel nails, standard polish, and natural nails on the hands of health care workers," *American Journal of Infection Control* 46, vol. 12 (2018): 1356–59, http://doi.org/10.1016/j.ajic.2018.05.022

Notes

1. "CDC's Core Infection Prevention and Control Practices for Safe Healthcare Delivery in All Settings," April 12, 2024, Centers for Disease Control and Prevention, https://www.cdc.gov/infection-control/hcp/core-practices/index.html.
2. Bryan Bledsoe et al., "EMS Provider Compliance with Infection Control Recommendations Is Suboptimal," *Prehospital Emergency Care* 18, no. 2 (2014): 290–4, https://doi.org/10.3109/10903127.2013.851311.
3. Joshua Bucher et al., "Handwashing Practices Among Emergency Medical Service Personnel", *Western Journal of Emergency Medicine* 16, vol. 5 (2015): 727–35, http://doi.org/10.5811/westjem.2015.7.25917.

4

Exposure Issues in the Community Paramedicine and Mobile-Integrated Health Work Setting

Defining Exposures

Bloodborne Exposure Defined

- Contaminated sharps injury
- Blood or other potentially infection materials that enters the eye, nose, or mouth
- Blood or OPIM in direct contact with nonintact skin
- Cuts with sharps objects covered with blood or other potentially infection materials

Other Potentially Infectious Materials

- Cerebrospinal fluid
- Synovial fluid
- Pleural fluid
- Pericardial fluid
- Peritoneal fluid
- Amniotic fluid

Body Fluids Which DO NOT Pose A Risk Unless They Contain Visible Blood

- Stool
- Sputum
- Tears

- Sweat
- Vomitus
- Saliva
- Urine
- Vaginal secretions and semen (only a risk through sexual contact)

Postexposure Procedures in Home Care

Postexposure procedures in home care situations create challenges that differ from the emergency care situation. In the home care situation, the designated infection control officer (DICO) will not be working with the emergency room physician because the patient is not transported. In this case, the DICO will be working directly with the patient's attending physician. This will require the development of new procedures for postexposure medical follow up and source patient testing. The patient's attending physician will have very specific information on the health status of the patient and will be the person to order source patient testing.

Scope of Practice

Obtaining source patient blood for postexposure testing will depend on the scope of practice for paramedics and EMTs. Is drawing blood within the scope of practice in your program? A study published in *Prehospital Emergency Care* in 2019 determined that there is a lack of guidance and consistency regarding community paramedicine (CP) programs and scope of practice. The study's authors reviewed programs across the country and determined that "it was not clear that state oversight of scope of practice for paramedics provides clear guidance of the novel functions and skills performed by CP programs."[1]

There are many different types of CP and mobile-integrated healthcare (MIH) programs across the country; some of them conduct wellness visits, some ensure that the community is up to date on vaccinations, and others perform more direct patient care activities. In any of these program types, the opportunity for exposure exists. In a vaccine and immunization program, for example, a contaminated needlestick injury might occur. In the home wellness visit situation, there could be an exposure to an airborne or droplet-transmitted disease involving the patient or a family member. A more probable situation in which an exposure might occur would be in the provision of more direct in-home care (i.e., managing direct intravenous site care and management).

Bloodborne Exposures

This is where scope of practice becomes important. Who can obtain the source patient's blood for testing? The Centers for Disease Control published a statement addressing emergency medical service personnel obtaining source patient blood. "[emergency medical service should not be involved in source patient testing. This is the responsibility of the medical facility and state human immunodeficiency virus testing laws do not state that this can be performed by other than the medical facility."[2]

That raises the question—what about using an oral swab for testing? The Center for Disease Control addressed this issue as well in the same published statement, stating that, "the oral swab test is NOT the acceptable test for source patient testing. Blood testing is the appropriate method. This is because the level of antibodies in oral fluid is lower than it is in blood; oral fluid tests find infection longer after exposure than do blood tests. Up to 1 in 12 infected people may test false-negative with this test. And, if a test shows positive results, repeat blood testing would need to follow."

Through consultation with a clinician at the PEP Hotline, a procedure was developed to assist with obtaining source patient testing in the home care environment. Discussion began with affirming that the DICO should be the person notified in an exposure situation, and they are responsible for contacting the patient's attending physician for patient history and orders for testing, if needed.

It was also decided that the DICO is responsible for conducting the source patient's testing. The type of testing method depends on the health history of the patient. If the patient is deemed to be low risk for having a bloodborne pathogen disease, then rapid fingerstick testing would be appropriate. The DICO would receive training on the use of rapid test kits and have them available if needed.

Rapid testing is available for human immunodeficiency virus, hepatitis C virus, and syphilis. These tests can be performed because they are waived under a Medicare and Medicaid amendment called the Clinical Laboratory Improvement Amendment (CLIA). In order for a rapid test to receive a CLIA waiver, it must be reviewed by the Food and Drug Administration and shown to be simple and have a low risk of error.

A CLIA waiver certificate must be obtained by the CP or MIH program in order for rapid tests to be performed. This task would be the responsibility of the medical director for the program. Once a CLIA waiver is granted, then rapid testing can be performed.[3]

Currently, there is not a rapid test in the United States for hepatitis B. There is one in Europe, and an effort is underway to make it available here. Most emergency medical service personnel have received the hepatitis B vaccine and should be protected. If that is not the case, then blood would need to be drawn to test for hepatitis B in unvaccinated (or unprotected) personnel. Again, scope of practice is important.

If rapid testing is negative, the DICO will inform the attending physician, followed by the exposed employee. Negative rapid tests eliminate the need for additional testing of the exposed employee.

Figure 4–1 is a sample of a flow chart which illustrates the procedure for follow-up for a low-risk patient exposure.

Figure 4–2 illustrates a sample procedure for follow-up involving a high-risk patient. A high-risk patient would be one that is known to be infected with a bloodborne pathogen disease or is in a high-risk group. In this case, venipuncture blood would need to be drawn. Once again, this would be done by the DICO if scope of practice permits and arrangements were made with a local laboratory to test the blood.

This testing would involve viral load testing, which will determine if the patient has any of the viruses circulating in their blood. The presence of a viral load would indicate the potential for disease transmission. This would then require that the exposed employee receive baseline testing and additional testing as indicated in the Centers for Disease Control guidelines which the Occupational Safety and Health Administration (OSHA) enforces.

The department will need to establish a direct bill system with the laboratory for the testing on the patient. OSHA states that the patient should not be

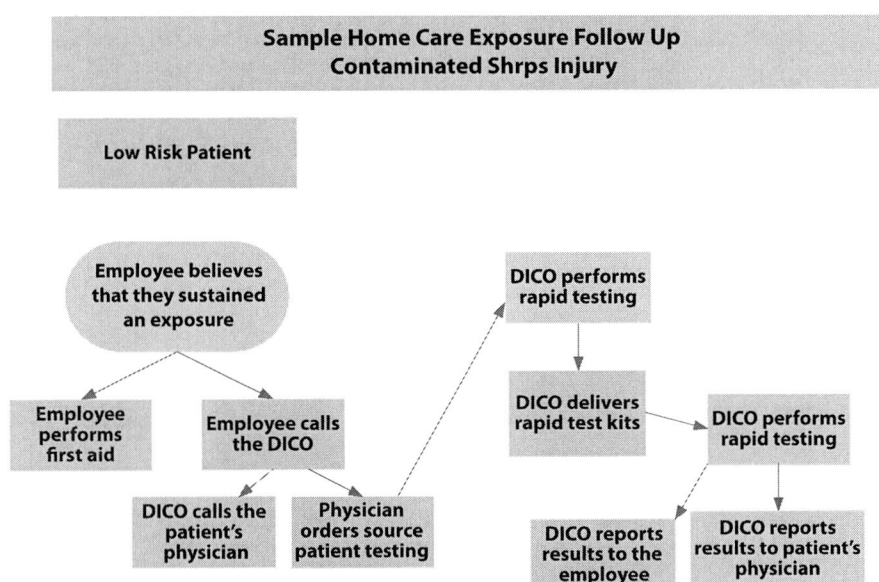

Figure 4–1. Follow-up for a low-risk patient exposure

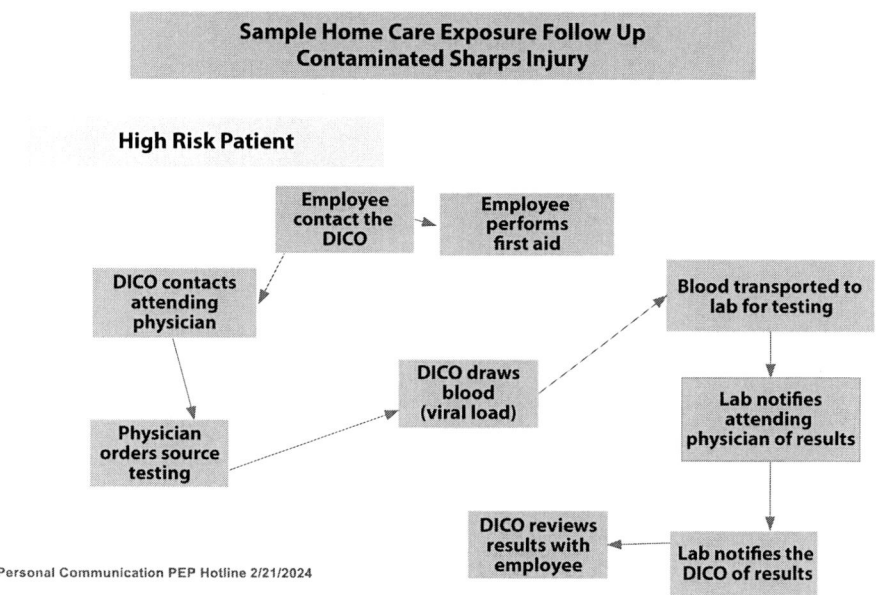

Figure 4–2. Follow-up for a high-risk patient exposure

charged for testing performed for the benefit of an exposed employee.[4] There are two states with exceptions to this requirement: South Carolina and New York.

If your CP and MIH program has a registered nurse on staff, then they can perform the testing, as that would be within their scope of practice.[5]

Airborne and Droplet Exposures

The procedure for notification and follow-up is very different because the notification will most likely come from the Public Health Department or the patient's attending physician. This is the procedure outlined in the Ryan White Act, as well as by OSHA. Notification is required if the patient is suspect for or diagnosed with an airborne or droplet transmitted disease. The point of contact will be the DICO.[6] The DICO will determine if an exposure occurred and make any needed referral for treatment with the designated medical provider for the department.

Notes

1. Melody Glenn et al., "State Regulation of Community Paramedicine Programs: A National Analysis," *Prehospital Emergency Care* 22, no. 22 (2017): 244–51.

2. Statement to Emergency Medical Services personnel regarding patient blood draws,, Centers for Disease Control and Prevention.
3. Barbara Phillips, "CLIA Waivers & Your Practice," February 21, 2021, Nurse Practitioner Business Owner, https://npbusiness.org/clia-waivers.
4. Enforcement Procedures for the Occupational Exposure to Bloodborne Pathogens, CPL 02-02-069 (2001).
5. Katherine West, "Post Exposure Medical Follow Up is Different in Mobile Integrated Health/Community Paramedicine Work," *Online Journal of Emergency Medical Services* (JEMS), April 26, 2024, https://www.jems.com/mobile-integrated-health-and-community-paramedicine/post-exposure-mobile-integrated-health-community-paramedicine/.
6. Ryan White Comprehensive AIDS Resources Emergency (CARE) Act, Pub. L. No. 101–308, 104 Stat. 576 (1990).

Basic Personal Protective Equipment in Home Care

Basic personal protective equipment (PPE) for home care includes the following:

- Disposable nonsterile gloves
- Sterile gloves in some instances such as dressing changes
- Utility or dishwashing style gloves (washable and reusable)
- Environmental Protection Agency-registered disinfectants
- Bleach and water at 1:100 dilution, mixed fresh daily (¼ cup bleach to one gallon of water)
- Cover gown
- Protective eyewear
- Waterless, alcohol-based hand cleaner
- Respiratory assist devices (disposable)

The Centers for Disease Control (CDC) published a guideline for the use of PPE for public safety services personnel. This serves as a great reference for a practical, science-based approach to the use of PPE. As illustrated, there has never been the need for the use of gloves for all patient contact. Use of PPE is based on the task being performed and contact with blood or other potentially infectious material. In the provision of home care, the need for glove use is generally lower than in the provision of emergent care. The provision of care in the home is a more controlled environment than an emergency care situation. Caring for a trauma patient with extensive injuries would require the use of multiple PPE items, but to perform a wound dressing change in the home situation would only require the use of gloves (table 5–1).

> Please note that gloves are *not* needed for all patient contact. This is clearly published by the CDC and the Occupational Safety and Health Administration (OSHA) in the bloodborne pathogens regulation. These would be frequent practices in the home care environment (table 5–2).

Table 5–1. Task-based PPE use from the CDC's Guide for Public Safety Personnel

Task	Gloves	Eyewear/Mask	Gown
Drawing blood	X	None	None
Decon equipment or surfaces	Utility style	If splatter or splash is anticipated	If splatter or splash is anticipated
Wound care	X	If splatter or splash is anticipated	If splatter or splash is anticipated
Injection	None	None	None
Intubation	X	X	Available
Delivery	X	X	X
IV site care	X	None	None
IV start	X	If splatter or splash is anticipated	Available
Monitors	None	None	None
Providing oxygen	None	None	None
Suctioning	X	Available	Available
Trauma	X	X	X
Vital signs	None	None	None
Foley catheter care	X	None	None

Table 5–2. Latex and nitrile glove allergy and sensitivity

Procedure	Rationale/Action
All staff and clients need to be asked about latex allergies or sensitivities.	OSHA, CDC, and NIOSH have all addressed the risk of latex allergies and sensitivities in healthcare workers and the general public.
Nitrile gloves are now also being associated with allergic reactions. Nitrile gloves have the same accelerators as latex, and some care providers are allergic to the color dyes in the gloves.	
Allergic patients or staff must be provided latex free equipment or care. For staff identified with allergy: • Obtain documentation of allergy history • Conduct an environmental survey • Refer to allergist • Provide safe alternatives to latex products • Evaluate the need for temporary or permanent work restrictions	Each employer of healthcare workers needs to address this issue to reduce the incidence of developing allergies, sensitivities, or a server reaction due to contact with latex or nitrile.
Create a latex free care environment.	Liability reduction and risk management.

Transmission-Based Precautions

When caring for a patient with a known infection, precautions for the healthcare provider are based on how the illness is transmitted. This is known as *transmission-based precaution*. This terminology applies to bloodborne, airborne, and droplet-transmitted diseases. Precautions include standard, contact, droplet, and airborne precautions.

Standard Precautions

The term *standard precautions* replaced *universal precautions and body substance isolation* in 2005.

- Assume blood and body fluid of *any* patient could be infectious (except sweat).
- Recommends PPE and other infection-control practices to prevent transmission in any healthcare setting.
- Decisions about PPE use are determined by the type of clinical interaction had with patients (task-based).

    ♦ This supports that gloves are *not* needed for all patient contact.

- **Gloves**—Use when touching blood, body fluids, secretions, excretions, contaminated items, mucus membranes, and nonintact skin.
- **Gowns**—Use during procedures and patient care activities when contact of clothing or exposed skin with blood or bodily fluids, secretions, or excretions is anticipated.
- **Mask and goggles** or a **face shield**—Use during patient care activities likely to generate splashes or sprays of blood, body fluids, secretions, or excretions.

Contact Precautions

- Designed to reduce the risk of transmission for organisms spread by direct or indirect contact.
- Recommends a gown if clothing may become soiled with patient secretion or excretions.
- Clean and disinfect all contact items, including the blood pressure cuff, stethoscope, and items that were in contact and used in the care of the patient. These are *high-touch surfaces*.

The following diseases necessitate contact precautions:

- Norovirus
- Multidrug resistant organisms
- Skin and wound infections
- Head lice
- Ebola
- COVID-19

Special Note: PPE for Ebola was downgraded for emergency medical services (EMS) in December of 2014.

Droplet Precautions

Droplet precautions are designed to reduce transmission of diseases involving medium to large size droplets. These droplets can travel three feet and drop to the floor.

Always use the following standard precautions:

- Place a surgical mask on the patient if you are within three feet; if it is not possible to place on the patient, place on yourself.
- Good handwashing protocol.

Diseases transmitted by droplets include the following:

- Influenza
- Pertussis (whooping cough)
- Meningitis
- Mumps
- Ebola
- Middle East respiratory syndrome (MERS)
- Avian-H5N1 (bird flu)

Airborne Precautions

Airborne precautions are designed to reduce transmission of illnesses carried by large particles which are dispersed by air currents. Fire and EMS should always follow the standard precaution of using a surgical mask within six feet.

The following diseases are covered under airborne precautions:

- Tuberculosis
- Chickenpox
- Measles

The CDC is in the process of updating their isolation guidelines. These guidelines were last updated in 2007.

The update will focus on a more scientific view of how infections are transmitted. The CDC has asked the Healthcare Infection Control Practices Advisory Committee to work on the updates. This is an independent group that makes recommendations to the CDC. Their update will be accomplished in stages. The first stage was to be completed by the end of June 2024 but has been delayed.[1]

Cleaning Patient Care Equipment

Patient care equipment which is not dedicated to the care of a specific patient must be cleaned after each patient use. This would include blood pressure cuffs, stethoscopes, and temperature monitors. Cleaning is essential in reducing the risk of cross-infection.

When considering an approach in the home care situation, consideration must be given to keeping the process simple and keeping the cost low. Costly hospital-level solutions are not necessary in the home care environment. It is also important to conduct cost–benefit analysis regarding the use of disposable items as opposed to reusable items.

The basic concept of cleaning and disinfection is that manual cleaning needs to be performed in order to achieve disinfection. Organic material interferes with achieving disinfection. Oftentimes, sales personnel will state that their product will kill everything, but it is well documented that cleaning is the essential first step! A published review of cleaning of EMS equipment showed that compliance with cleaning equipment was low.[2]

In a Duke University study, it was noted that stethoscopes were cleaned only about 4% of the time. The responders in the survey also stated that stethoscopes were not disinfected at all about 82% of the time. It also noted that vehicles were cleaned about 33–55% of the time.[3]

Another systematic review was conducted regarding the cleaning of stethoscopes. It involved a review of 253 publications. Studies show that about 32% of healthcare-associated infections were preventable. It was noted in the studies that handwashing and improper disinfection of medical devices was a main source for infection transmission. It is specifically noted that stethoscopes were rarely disinfected properly and could result in cross infection.[4]

Stethoscopes and blood pressure cuffs are listed as noncritical items, as they are in direct contact with intact skin. Based on this, the CDC states that blood pressure cuffs can be cleaned using a detergent and should be cleaned before and after each use.

Stethoscopes should be cleaned after each use.[5] Isopropyl alcohol and sodium hypochlorite have been shown to be effective for cleaning them. Stethoscopes have been implicated in the transfer of bacterial infections.[6]

General surface cleaning in the home care environment can be performed using commonly found items such as ammonia, baking soda, or vinegar. Vinegar has been used as a disinfectant agent for centuries.

Notes

1. Daniel Jernigan and John Howard, "A CDC Update on the Part One Draft Update to the Guideline for Isolation Precautions: Preventing Transmission of Infectious Agents in Healthcare Settings," Centers for Disease Control and Prevention, 2024.
2. Diego Schaps, et al., "Medical Transport-Associated Infection: Review and Commentary Making a Case for Its Legitimacy," *Infection Control & Hospital Epidemiology* 43, no. 4 (2022): 497–503, https://doi.org/10.1017/ice.2020.1354.
3. Gabriele Messina et al., "Tanning the Bugs—A Pilot Study of an Innovative Approach to Stethoscope Disinfection," *Journal of Hospital Infection*, vol. 95 (2017): 228–230, https://doi.org/10.1016/j.jhin.2016.12.005.
4. Margherita Napolitani et al. "Methods of Disinfecting Stethoscopes: Systematic Review," *International Journal of Environmental Research and Public Health* 17, no. 6 (2020): 1856, https://doi.org/10.3390/ijerph17061856.
5. "Disinfection in Ambulatory Care, Home Care, and the Home," *Guideline for Disinfection and Sterilization in Healthcare Facilities* (Centers for Disease Control and Prevention, 2008).
6. José Reginaldo Alves de Queiroz Junior, et al. "Identification and Resistance Profile of Bacteria Isolated on Stethoscopes by Healthcare Professionals: Systematic Review," *American Journal of Infection Control* 49, no. 2 (2021): 229–237, https://doi.org/10.1016/j.ajic.2020.07.007.

Patient Care Infection Control and General Health

Care of a patient in the community paramedicine (CP) or mobile-integrated healthcare (MIH) program begins with a review of the patient's medical record from the medical facility. The discharge summary is key to assessing the patient's care needs.

The medical facility should have discharge planners who assist in establishing a plan to facilitate the patient's recovery after discharge. The discharge summary and plan can help with patient and family education and prevent readmissions. It is well known that the educational component of patient discharge falls on the nursing staff. Recent studies have shown that is not optimal due to issues of time constraints and staffing shortages. Other factors noted have been language barriers, high-risk environments, and lack of medication management. These factors have been found to account for 30% of hospital admissions and readmissions. When this component is missing in the discharge process, readmission may be the result. Readmissions are costly and result in a negative experience for the patient and their family.[1]

CP and MIH care providers need appropriate discharge summaries and plans to assist in the provision of optimum care.[2] Physician orders for in-home care need to be closely reviewed and coordinated with the patient's attending physician and the home care providers.

Some key information is needed from the discharge summary, such as current medications (cost and access) and contact for the primary care physician. Food security is also important. How will the patient access food?

Maintaining the patient's ongoing medical record will be a new task and responsibility for emergency medical services (EMS) providers. The maintenance of patient medical information is an important part of care and legal liability reduction. Tables 6-1 and 6-2 are designed to assess patient care needs.

When assigned to a patient, it is important to not only review the patient's medical discharge records, but also to access the home situation for safety and potential additional care needs. The following forms are designed to assist in

Table 6–1. Basic infection control: assessing patient's dwelling posthospital discharge (Document process and all procedures for confidential patient records.)[16]

Procedure	Rationale/Action
Complete a visual inspection of dwelling.	Notify patient's case worker of potential health hazards.
Assess dwelling's general cleanliness.	Potential infection source
Assess dwelling floor plan.	Patient's ease of movement Potential trip and fall hazards Medications are easily accessible to patient
Assess dwelling for infestations of • Bed bugs • Roaches • Rodents	Potential infection sources • Presence of bites on patient • Presence of bug bombs or insecticide sprays • Evidence of smashed bugs on the walls • Evidence of feces or droppings • Mouse traps or sticky traps
When entering dwelling with suspected infestation • Spray DEET on shoes and pants • Limit items taken into the dwelling • Place items in plastic bin • Place dressing materials into plastic bags	Schedule visits to this dwelling last.

the process of conducting a home safety and needs evaluation. When completed, these forms should be a part of the patient's ongoing medical record. Any additional needs should be reported to the patient's case manager or physician.[3]

As healthcare professionals pursue the discussion of acute hospital to home care, even more policies and procedures will need to be developed. The model for this approach to delivering acute patient care in the home situation comes from Australia and Great Britain. This model has now been tested by the John Hopkins Schools of Medicine and Public Health 1995, and focuses on older adults, persons with chronic conditions, and those with multiple comorbidities. This model has become described as the next generation of health care. This approach has been shown to be cost effective, and patients report an increased sense of well-being, which promotes patient safety and quality of care. In the testing phase, patients expressed great satisfaction with the program.[4] However, this will require more training and education for families that will be involved in the care of their loved ones. Infection prevention will need to be a strong focus in this training to prevent posthospital infections and patient readmission.

Reviewing the patient's medical record is vital to assessing the patient's care needs. This chapter contains a sample summary from a medical facility. Physician orders concerning care in the home environment should follow. A close review and coordination of patient care needs should be established. The

Table 6–2. CP or MIH home care safety checklist

Patient Name: _____ Discharge Date: _____ Date: _____

Criteria	Compliance YES	Compliance NO	Observation/Notes
Living Area			
Does the room have adequate lighting?			
Is there a clear walkway?			
Are throw rugs present?			
Are there electrical cords or extensions in foot traffic area?			
Do the stairs have a sturdy handrail?			
Do the stairs have adequate lighting?			
Kitchen Area			
Does the room have adequate lighting?			
Are dishes and glassware at an accessible level?			
Will a step stool be needed to access dishes and glassware?			
Bathroom Area			
Does the room have adequate lighting?			
Is a toilet raiser needed?			
Does the tub or shower have a slip-free mat?			
Does the tub or shower have grab bars?			
Does the tub or shower need grab bars?			
Is a shower seat present?			
Is a shower seat needed?			
Bedroom Area			
Does the room have adequate lighting?			
Is there a light switch accessible from the bed?			
Is there a phone near the bed?			
Is there a clear pathway to the bathroom?			
Is there a night light present?			
Home Overview			
General cleanliness is good			
Infestations noted			
Corrective Action Plan 1. 2. 3. 4. 5.			

maintenance of patient medical information is an important part of care and legal liability reduction (tables 6–1 and 6–2).[5]

After assessment, focus then needs to be placed on an extensive review of the patient's discharge summary from the medical facility. Make notes of any allergies or additional supplies needed for patient care. This is a new responsibility for EMS personnel and will require some additional preparation and awareness of area resources (table 6–3).

Evaluation of the patient's understanding of any prescribed medications and possible mobility restrictions need to be reviewed with the patient or family members who will be assisting in the patient's care. The following procedure is to assist in the process of discharging a patient with a medical diagnosis.[6]

The following procedure is designed to assist in the evaluation of a patient discharged with postdischarge surgical care needs (table 6–4).

Recording the appearance of the postsurgical wound area is an essential part of documentation that may impact identification of an infection noted on discharge. This would also affect the medical facility's healthcare infection rate. These rates are generally procedure-based and are required to be reported. Finally, assess the family's need for education and training if they will be participating in the care of the patient and their surgical wound site.[7]

Table 6–3. Assessing patient's status posthospital medical discharge (Document process and all procedures for confidential patient records)

Procedure	Rationale/Action
Complete a patient medical assessment.	
Obtain medical history.	Identify needs related to medical history, such as • Medical allergies • Medical supply allergies
Check patient vital signs.	
Assess patient's mobility needs.	Assist with additional needs for a walker, cane, etc.
Review patient discharge instructions.	Assess patient's understanding.
Review hospital discharge plan.	Discharge planner may have referrals or follow up prescriptions.
Review medications with patient.	Ensure patient's understanding of medication instructions such as the • Time to be taken • Special instructions (taken before, with, or after meals)
Assess family's understanding of patient's care needs by reviewing patient's discharge instructions.	Assess understanding of patient's needs.

The transition from emergency care to home care requires a review of new terminology. Listed here are two key terms that will be used in the provision of home care (table 6–5). Use of proper terminology is important in being recognized as a member of the healthcare team.[8]

Table 6–4. Assessing patient's status posthospital surgical discharge (Document process and all procedures for confidential patient records)

Procedure	Rationale/Action
Complete a patient medical assessment.	
Assess patient's mobility needs.	Assist with additional needs: • Walker, cane, etc.
Check patient vital signs.	
Assess surgical site and observe for fever, signs of redness, or swelling.	Document appearance of wound.
If noted • Notify surgeon • Notify infection preventionist	Postoperative infections are to be reported to the medical facility and the facility will report to CMS.
Review hospital discharge instructions.	Assess patient's understanding.
Review medications with patient.	Ensure patient's understanding of medication instructions such as • Time to be taken • Special instructions (taken before, with, or after meals)
Assess family's understanding of patient's care needs by reviewing patient's discharge instructions.	Assess understanding of patient's needs.

Table 6–5. Clarifying terms for home care

Aseptic Technique
Aseptic technique is utilized to maximize and maintain asepsis, or the absence of pathogenic organisms, in the clinical setting. The goals of aseptic technique are to protect the patient from infection and to prevent the spread of pathogens. In health care, aseptic techniques deter infection when working with patients. For example, when doing IV site prep, work in a circular motion from the site outward—never return to the site.
Clean Technique
In the nonhospital setting, *clean technique* involves reducing the numbers of microorganisms to minimize the risk of transmission from the environment or healthcare personnel, using the appropriate hand hygiene and clean gloves.
Paramedics will use clean technique in the home care setting.

Caring for Patients with Multidrug-Resistant Infections

If a patient presents with a documented multidrug-resistant infection, the patient should be scheduled as the last patient of the day. Items used to care for the patient such as the blood pressure cuff and the stethoscope should only be used for that patient.

It is not uncommon for EMS to be unaware that a patient has an infection due to a multidrug-resistant organism. It would be beneficial to work with medical facilities in your area and long-term care facilities to establish an interagency communication agreement to ensure that you receive notification. A proper care schedule and proper cleaning and disinfection solutions as well as handwash solutions can be made available. This is important to prevent cross-infection.

Caring for a postoperative surgical wound is a new task for EMS personnel which requires specific training, such as screening the patient's surgical area for signs of infection and properly dressing that area. Wound assessment is important as documentation of a possible postdischarge infection can create the need for additional reporting to the medical facility and attending physician (table 6–6).

Table 6–6. Dressing change: observing for signs of infection in a surgical wound (Document process and all procedures for confidential patient records)

Procedure	Rationale/Action
Check vital signs.	Check for elevated temperature.
Check if patient received wound care discharge instructions.	Review wound care instructions.
Wash hands.	Use soap and water for basic infection control.
Put on gloves.	Use standard precautions for basic infection control.
Remove dressing.	
Observe for redness, swelling, odor, pain, or drainage at wound site.	Document wound appearance.
Place dressing materials in a regular trash bag.	Dressing materials are not considered medical waste in home care.
Wash hands.	
Clean wound.	Use saline solution or soapy water.
Wipe easy to remove dried blood or drainage around incision.	Reduces risk of infection.
Apply new dressing.	Check if an ointment is advised or a new type of dressing.
Wash hands.	Always wash hands after patient care and glove removal.

EMS personnel are very proficient at starting an IV in the field, but starting an IV in the home situation is a bit different (tables 6–7 and 6–8).

Table 6–7. IV site insertion (Document process and all procedures for confidential patient records)

Procedure	Rationale/Action
In adults, use an upper-extremity site for catheter insertion.	
Avoid the use of steel needles.	They may cause tissue necrosis and extravasation.
Perform hand hygiene procedures: • Washing hands with soap and water • Alcohol-based hand rubs	Reduces possible infection
Prepare clean skin with an antiseptic (70% alcohol, tincture of iodine, iodophor, or chlorhexidine gluconate*) before peripheral venous catheter insertion.	Allow to dry before insertion for infection prevention.
Hand hygiene should be performed before and after • Palpating catheter insertion sites • Inserting, replacing, accessing, repairing, or dressing intravascular catheter	Basic infection control

*February 2017 Food and Drug Administration (FDA) warning: Healthcare professionals should always ask patients if they have ever had an allergic reaction to any antiseptic before recommending or prescribing a chlorhexidine gluconate product.

Table 6–8. Needle insertion technique (Document process and all procedures for confidential patient records)

Procedure	Rationale/Action
Wash hands.	
Palpate for vein selection.	
Apply tourniquet above the selected site.	For best results, place 3" above selected site. For patients with chronic obstructive pulmonary disease (COPD) or rolling veins, do *not* use a tourniquet.
Prep site with a chlorhexidine solution.	A 2% chlorhexidine solution offers an effective one-step prep. A new formulation eliminates the concern for allergies. Alcohol is not effective unless a one-minute friction rub is used. Prep should be done in a circular motion starting in the center and moving out.
Wear gloves.	Gloves should be worn if there is a chance of blood spillage.
Insert needle at a 45-degree angle.	For patients with COPD or rolling veins, bevel down technique is suggested.
Dispose of needle into a sharps container.	If a vacutainer is used, make sure the sharps container has a vacutainer adapter.

(continued)

Procedure	Rationale/Action
Wear clean gloves.	Sterile gloves are not required for peripheral IVs.
Use either sterile gauze or sterile, transparent, semipermeable dressing to cover the catheter site.	
Evaluate the catheter insertion site daily by palpation through the dressing to discern tenderness and by inspection if a transparent dressing in use.	Observe for infection.
Do *not* use topical antibiotic ointment or creams on insertion sites.	
Gauze and opaque dressings should *not* be removed if the patient has no clinical signs of infection.	Document on patient records and report.
If the patient has local tenderness, opaque dressing should be removed and the site inspected visually.	

Proper, well-established infection control procedures must be followed. An IV site or bloodstream infection resulting from improper technique would be a reportable event to the medical facility and to the attending physician.

An infection resulting from improper IV administration meets the definition of a healthcare-associated infection (HAI). These infections are being closely monitored, and so they must be reported to the medical facility who in turn reports to the Center for Medicare and Medical Services (CMS).

The following are policies and procedures for infection control practices in the home care situation applicable to IV infusion.[9]

Table 6–9 documents the procedure for care of the established IV site.

Table 6–9. IV peripheral site care (Document process and all procedures for confidential patient records; adapted from 2011 Centers for Disease Control [CDC] Guidelines)

Procedure	Rationale/Action
Inspect site daily.	Observe for signs of infection phlebitis or infiltration.
	Do not apply topical antibiotics or creams.
	Apply chlorhexidine-impregnated dressings (FDA cleared).
If signs of phlebitis are noted, notify physician.	Symptoms of phlebitis include redness, warmth, and pain in the affected area.

Procedure	Rationale/Action
Catheter *should* be removed; treatment orders may include warm compress, anti-inflammatory medication, compression stockings, and blood thinners.	
Perform hand hygiene.	Wash hands with soap and water or an alcohol-based hand cleaner.
Cleanse area using a 2% chlorhexidine wash. For short-term catheters: • Replace gauze dressing every 2 days. • Replace transparent dressing every 7 days.	
Apply clean gloves.	Sterile gloves are *not* required.
Remove dressing.	
Clean the area with 2% chlorhexidine.	Reduces the risk of catheter-related bloodstream infections. Observe for possible allergic reactions, wheezing or difficulty breathing, swelling of the face, hives that can quickly progress to other more serious symptoms, severe rash, and shock.[a]
Apply dressing to the site.	Use sterile gauze, or a sterile transparent, semipermeable dressing.
If patient is diaphoretic, use a gauze dressing.	
Needleless components • Change administration sets every 72 hours. • Change needleless connectors every 72 hours.	
Scrub access port with an antiseptic.	Infection prevention
Use needleless systems to access IV tubing.	
Do *not* apply topical antibiotic ointment or creams to the insertion site	May promote the growth of fungal infection and antimicrobial resistance.
Place dressing material in a bag.	Place in general trash, not medical waste.
Wash hands.	
There is no need to replace peripheral catheters more frequently than every 72–96 hours.	

[a] "FDA warns about rare but serious allergic reactions with the skin antiseptic chlorhexidine gluconate," U.S. Food and Drug Administration, 2017; "Proper Site Prep for Injections," World Health Organization, 2010.

Table 6–10 details site care for peripherally-inserted central catheters (PICCs). Table 6–11 details the procedures for bathing and perineal care.

Table 6–10. IV central line—PICC site care (Document process and all procedures for confidential patient records; adapted from 2011 CDC Guidelines)

Procedure	Rationale/Action
Use for longer than 6 days of intravascular therapy.	
Check with patient regarding discharge site care instructions.	Note on patient record.
Inspect site daily.	Observe for signs of infection, phlebitis or infiltration.
If signs of phlebitis are noted, notify physician.	Symptoms include redness, warmth, and pain in the affected area.
	PICC lines have been associated with higher risk for deep vein thrombosis and for blood stream infections.
Catheter should be removed; treatment orders may include warm compress, anti-inflammatory medication, compression stockings, and blood thinners.	
Check that the site is clean and dry.	Area should be covered with a waterproof cover (plastic wrap) when showering.
Perform hand hygiene.	Wash hands with soap and water or an alcohol-based hand cleaner.
Apply sterile or clean gloves.	
Clean the area with 0.5% chlorhexidine prep with alcohol.	Reduces the risk of catheter-related bloodstream infections.
Dispose of dressing material in a regular trash bag.	Dressing material is not considered medical waste in home care.

Table 6–11. Bathing and perineal care procedures

Procedure	Rationale/Action
Standardize time and procedure.	Make part of daily bathing
Perform after an incontinence event.	Prevent skin breakdown and infection
Apply 2% chlorhexidine gluconate solution.	Reduces risk of infection

One of the main issues in the home care situation is the maintenance of an indwelling urinary catheter. Improper maintenance is one of the leading causes of HAIs and patient readmissions. This is a new procedure for EMS providers and will require additional training (table 6–12).

Table 6–12. Foley catheter care for home care clients (Document process and all procedures for confidential patient records)[17]

Procedure	Rationale/Action
Use aseptic technique for insertion *only* when necessary.	Sterile equipment
Use standard precautions (good hand-washing and gloves).	Urinary tract infections (UTIs) are the leading cause of infection
Ensure the catheter is secured to the patient's leg or abdomen (see figure 6–1 for proper positioning).	This will assist in preventing movement, urethral traction, and bladder trauma.
Keep the urine collection bag below the level of the bladder.	Prevents backup of urine which can lead to infection
Maintain unobstructed urine flow	Infection prevention
Check for signs of infection	
Wash hands before and after handling catheter.	Infection prevention
Clean the area around the drainage tube twice each day.	
Use soap and water to carefully wash around the drainage tube.	
Rinse well and dry with a clean towel.	
Maintain a closed system.	Infection prevention
If opened, wipe with alcohol.	Infection prevention
Wipe at the catheter junction.	
Empty the bag regularly, use a container with measurement marks (see figure 6–2 for proper positioning).	Record output in patient record
Do not allow the drainage spigot to touch the container.	Prevention of cross-infection
Clean perineal area with mild soap and water and 2% chlorohexidine.	Infection prevention
Encourage good fluid intake.	Reduce incidence of infection

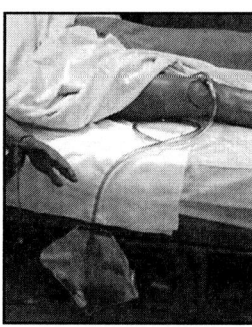

Figure 6–1. Closed urinary drainage. Patient should not lie on the tubing. The bag should be hung from the bedframe.

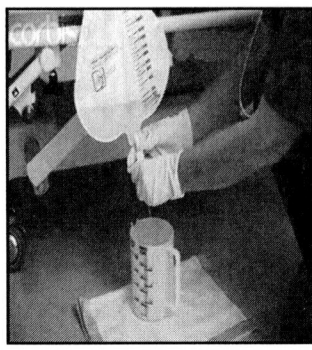

Figure 6–2. Emptying drainage bag

Currently, it is often the practice for EMS personnel transporting a patient with an indwelling urinary catheter to place the bag between the patient's legs on top of the stretcher for transport. This allows the possibility of urine backing up and could lead to a urinary tract infection (UTI). This would result in an HAI for which the medical facility may not be reimbursed.

Now that policies for urinary care have been addressed, it is important to examine additional surgical wound care issues. Many patients are returned to home care with a new ostomy or a tracheostomy. These will require an emotional adjustment involving a great deal of education and assistance for both the patient and family. EMS care providers will therefore require additional education and training (tables 6–13 and 6–14).

Table 6–13. Ostomy care (Document process and all procedures for confidential patient records; adapted from 2011 CDC Guidelines)[18]

Procedure	Rationale/Action
Ensure the patient has been properly fitted for the bag "punching system."	Proper fit prevents leakage and possible skin breakdown (See figure 6–3).
If leakage is noted, a new fitting is required.	
Access patient knowledge of what defines a full bag.	If the bag is over-filled, the bag will pull away from the skin.
	1/3 filled is considered full.
Conduct the change in the bathroom.	
Wear gloves.	Infection prevention
Cleanse the area with soap and water.	Dry well.
Apply new pouch, and make sure that the hole is as close to the stoma as possible.	Protects the skin
The "punching system" should be changed in the morning before breakfast.	The intestinal system is less active in the morning.
Change at least every 3 days.	If there is more liquid, change more frequently.

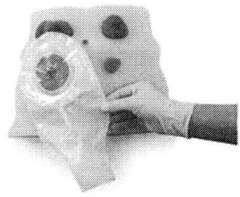

Figure 6–3. Bag placement on an ostomy site

Table 6–14. Tracheostomy care (Document process and all procedures for confidential patient records)[19]

Procedure	Rationale/Action
Routine tracheostomy care should be done at least once a day after discharge (figure 6–4)	Infection prevention
Consider a clean procedure, if less than one month old consider a sterile procedure	
Wash your hands with soap and water	
Put on gloves	
Suction the trach tube	Clear secretions
Disinfect the inner cannula by pouring over with hydrogen peroxide (figure 6–5)	
Clean out and dry with a pipe cleaner	
Rinse with normal saline, tap water or distilled water.	
Reinsert the cannula and lock in place.	
Inspect for signs of infection, such as redness, swelling, odor, or tenderness.	
Soak cotton swab in half hydrogen peroxide and half water solution for cleaning.	Infection prevention
Dry exterior area with clean cloth.	
Clean off the hydrogen peroxide solution.	
Change trach ties.	
Place mesh gauge under trach tie.	Do *not* use gauze or toppers as cotton fibers may clog the airway.
Remove gloves.	Discard in general trash, as they are not medical waste in home care.
Wash hands.	Important after glove removal

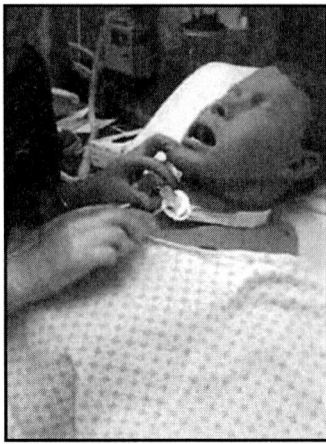

Figure 6–4. Cleaning of the tracheostomy site

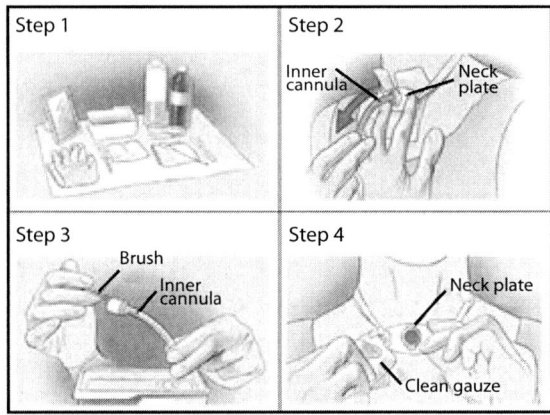

Figure 6–5. Cleaning the inner cannula

Assessment for Diabetic Foot Ulcers

Care of feet for a diabetic requires a multidisciplinary approach (table 6–15). Home care plays a vital role in this assessment and management. Assessment includes monitoring vascular, metabolic, and microbiological aspects as well as an educational focus for the patient and family members (figs. 6–6 and 6–7). Dishwashing-style gloves are washable and reusable. Their use also lowers cost.[10]

Caring for Your Feet

Keep your feet protected and healthy to prevent open sores and wounds on your feet.

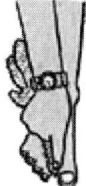
Keep your feet clean and dry.

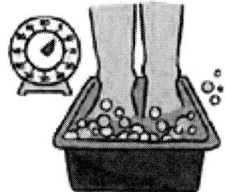
Do not soak your feet for a long time.

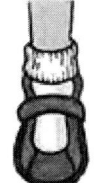
Wear clean socks every day and always wear shoes with a closed toe and heel.

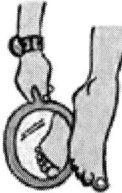
Check your feet daily for blisters, redness or sores. See your doctor right away if you have any sores.

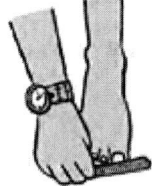
Routinely use an emery board to trim nails. Never use a razor or a knife.

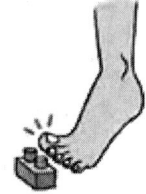
Keep floors and paths clear of objects to avoid stubbing your toes.

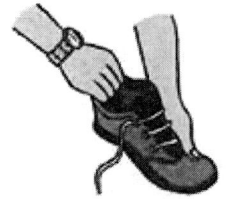
Examine your shoes every day.

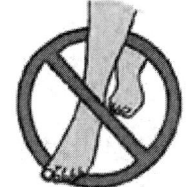
Never walk barefoot or wear flip flops.

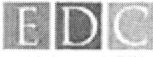

Figure 6-6. Caring for your feet[20,21]

Infection Control Policies for Community Paramedicine and MIH

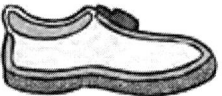

How to Pick the Right Shoe

When you shop for shoes, take this tip sheet with you.
Take your time to carefully select shoes. You are looking for a shoe that protects your feet, keeps them dry and offers support as you walk.

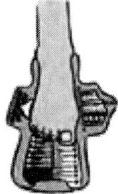

- Have your foot measured to make sure you are selecting the right size and width.

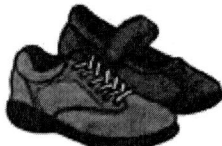

- Select a shoe with flexible fittings, such as laces or "hook and loop" straps. Avoid slip ons.

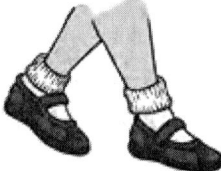

- Try on the shoes with socks and walk in them at the store.
- Pay attention to the fit. No part of the shoe should pinch your feet.

- The inside should be smooth and have no seams.
- Look for cushioned insole that prevents rubbing or friction.
- The ankle area should be soft and supportive.

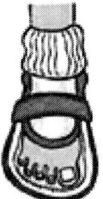

- The toe box should be wide enough so you can wiggle your toes.
- Your foot should not slide inside the shoe as you walk.

Everyone with Diabetes Counts

Figure 6–7. How to pick the right shoe

Table 6–15. Assessment for diabetic foot ulcers

Procedure	Rationale/Action
Monitor blood glucose levels.	
Monitor blood pressure.	Adequate circulation is important. Patient should *not* smoke.
Visual assessment: • Physical assessment of feet at risk • Assessment of pulses • Sensory exam (touch, vibrations, monofilament) • Check nails for trimming	
• Check for need for debridement	Dead tissue is a breeding ground for bacteria.
Teach proper foot care.	Proper footwear (ask about neuropathy)
Observe for callus.	Can lead to ulceration (if noted, alert treating physician)

General Cleaning

The importance of proper cleaning and disinfection routines should not be new to EMS care providers; in fact, the manner in which these are conducted will be the same in many ways. The basic disinfectant, bleach and water at a 1:100 dilution, is the same. Focusing on high-touch items is also the same. It is important to note, however, that the Occupational Safety and Health Administration (OSHA) requires dishwashing-style gloves to be used—not latex or nitrile (table 6–16).[11]

Some patients in home care may be prescribed to use a humidifier. The following is a procedure for cleaning this device to prevent the possible development of a respiratory infection (table 6–17).[12]

Some patients in home care may be prescribed to use a glucose-monitoring device. The following is a procedure for cleaning this device (table 6–18).

Razors and Fingerstick Pens

The proper handling and disposal of sharps in the home situation is important, especially if the patient has a bloodborne pathogen illness. OSHA defers to the individual state's medical waste regulation for disposal. Most of these regulations permit sharps to be disposed of in the general trash if first placed into a coffee can or plastic detergent bottle. This is a major difference in sharps disposal in the home situation (table 6–19).

Table 6–16. Routine surface cleaning (Document process and all procedures for confidential patient records)

Procedure	Rationale/Action
Use dishwashing-style gloves for all cleaning activities.	OSHA required, inexpensive, washable, and reusable
Surfaces in bathroom and shower are to be cleaned after use, if contaminated, and on a once-weekly basis.	Reduce the risk of cross-infection
Use a solution of bleach to water at 1:100 (1/4 cup bleach to 1 gallon of water) or Lysol concentrate 2 ½ tsp. per gallon of water)	EPA approved solutions A chlorine-based cleaning solution is needed to kill organisms such as C. diff, norovirus or C. auris
Clean areas and rinse with water.	
Discard solutions after 24 hours.	OSHA requirement, solutions lose effectiveness after that time
Wash off gloves and hang them to dry.	

Table 6–17. Cleaning humidifiers (Document process and all procedures for confidential patient records)

Procedure	Rationale/Action
All respiratory equipment should be thoroughly cleaned between uses with plain soap and water.	Cleaning is the key first step to achieving disinfection.
The unit should then be disinfected by using a liquid chemical agent which is EPA approved.	EPA is the regulatory agency for the approval of cleaning and disinfecting solutions.
Lysol disinfection meets these requirements (diluted at 2 ¼ tsp. per gallon of water).	OSHA requirement for chemical use
Wash down the unit and rinse with sterile water.	Tap water or distilled water may harbor microorganisms.
Dry and cover until next use.	

Table 6–18. Procedure for cleaning glucose-monitoring devices (Document process and all procedures for confidential patient records)[22]

Procedure	Rationale/Action
Fingerstick pens (reusable)	Have been linked to hepatitis B outbreaks
Never to be used for more than one person	
Use single-use lancets	Failure to change lancets, disposable platforms or endcaps between each patient
Auto-disabling fingerstick devices	Should be used (disposable)

Procedure	Rationale/Action
Dispose in sharps container	Sharps are medical waste
Blood glucose meters	
Assign to each person	
Wear gloves	Potential exposure to blood
Change gloves between each patient	Gloves are general trash
If shared, clean and disinfect after every use	Basic infection control practice
Follow the manufacturer's instructions	
Monitor compliance	Part of compliance monitoring
	Liability reduction and risk management

Table 6–19. Handling and disposal of razors (Document process and all procedures for confidential patient records)

Procedure	Rationale/Action
Each person is to have their own razor.	For sanitary reasons, razors should *not* be shared. Bloodborne diseases have been transmitted by the sharing of razors.
Used razors should be placed into a container for disposal in the general landfill.	Household razors are *not* considered medical waste.

Wound Irrigation

Many home care patients need wound irrigation. Table 6–20 outlines the performance procedure for infection control.[13]

Table 6–20. Solutions for irrigation (Document process and all procedures for confidential patient records)

Procedure	Rationale/Action
Irrigation solutions • Normal saline • Dakin's solution • Acetic acid (white vinegar)	
Discard within 1 week of opening.	Prevent contamination of solutions
Date the bottle when opened.	
Store in a cool place away from direct sunlight.	Slows growth of infectious organisms

Specimen Transport to Lab

Both OSHA and the CDC state that specimens transported and sent for laboratory evaluation should be handled in a specific manner. The following table explains that procedure (table 6–21).

Table 6–21. Transport of specimens (Document process and all procedures for confidential patient records)

Procedure	Rationale/Action
All specimens (blood, urine, stool) should be handled wearing vinyl gloves.	Although urine and stool do *not* pose a risk for the transmission of bloodborne pathogens, this is a good general rule.
Specimens to be sent to a lab for testing should be placed into a plastic bag and sealed.	This is to prevent spillage.
The plastic bag should have a biohazard label placed on it.	This is an OSHA requirement.
Once the specimen is sealed in the bag, remove gloves and wash hands.	Any soap is fine for handwashing.

Disposal of Discontinued Medications

In today's world, it is important to ensure that discontinued medications are properly disposed of to protect groundwater and to ensure that medications do not get into the hands of unauthorized persons. The disposal procedure is listed in table 6–22.[14]

Assessment of Patient Infection

The CDC and other infection-control groups have developed set criteria for assessing patient infections in the home care setting. It is important to review this information and to record infections in the patient's ongoing medical record. This will be new for EMS care providers and should therefore be included in education and training programs.

Most infections in the medical care setting are diagnosed by culture results. In the home care setting, however, visual inspection is the key practice. Here are some guidelines developed by the CDC to assist in the identification of possible infections. Home care providers should focus on the clinical data listing until laboratory data is available (table 6–23).

Table 6–22. Disposing of unused patient medications

Procedure	Rationale/Action
Follow any specific disposal instructions on the prescription drug labeling or patient information that accompanies the medicine.	Do *not* flush medications down the sink or toilet unless this specifically instructs that is to be done.
Utilize programs that allow the public to take unused drugs to a central location for proper disposal.	Call your local law enforcement agencies to see if they sponsor medicine take-back programs in your community. Contact the city's or county government's household trash and recycling service to learn about medication disposal options and guidelines.
If there are *no* programs in the area, remove them from their original containers and mix them with an undesirable substance, such as used coffee grounds, dirt, or kitty litter.	This makes the drug less appealing to children and pets, and unrecognizable to people who may intentionally go through the trash seeking drugs.
Place the mixture in a sealable bag, empty can, or other container to prevent the drug leaking or breaking out of a garbage bag.	
Scratch out all identifying information on the prescription label.	Privacy protection

Table 6–23. Assessment of Patient Infection

Criteria for Definitions of Home Health Care Infections		
Site of infection	Clinical data	Laboratory data
Catheter-related UTI		
	Change in characteristics of urine	Elevated serum leukocytes
	Fever	Evidence of UTI in urinalysis
	Pain	Evidence of leukocytes in urine dipstick test
		Positive urine culture (>105 CFU of a single organism per mL of urine)
Postoperative pneumonia		
	Change in character of sputum	Elevated serum leukocytes
	Decreased breath sounds	Sputum Gram stain smear with evidence of respiratory infection
	Increase in rales and rhonchi	
	Fever	Positive sputum culture
	Shortness of breath	Positive chest X-ray
	Pain	

(*continued*)

Criteria for Definitions of Home Health Care Infections		
Site of infection	Clinical data	Laboratory data
Catheter-related bloodstream infection		
	Fever with chills and rigors	Elevated serum leukocytes
	Redness, tenderness, or pain at insertion site	Positive blood culture
	Purulent drainage at site	Positive catheter culture (after catheter removal)
Skin and soft tissue infection		
	Pain, swelling, or tenderness at site	Gram stain smear with leukocytes and organisms
	Inflammation and warmth	Positive culture
	Purulent drainage	Elevated serum leukocytes
	Fever	
Endometritis in postpartum patients		
	Uterine tenderness and abdominal pain	Positive Gram stain smear of lochia
	Purulent vaginal drainage (lochia)	Positive culture of lochia
	Foul-smelling lochia	Remarkably elevated serum leukocytes
	Fever	

Definitions of Infection in Home Care Setting

Urinary Tract Infections

Symptomatic Urinary Tract Infections. Symptomatic urinary tract infections can occur without prior instrumentation (e.g., intermittent catheterization), but this is rare.

Catheter-Associated Urinary Tract Infections. Catheter-associated UTIs are associated with instrumentation of the patient's urinary tract prior to onset. To associate these infections with an indwelling urinary catheter requires presence of an indwelling urinary catheter at the time of or within 7 days before the onset of the symptomatic UTI.

Symptomatic and catheter-associated UTIs must meet one of the following criteria:

1. Two of the following four signs or symptoms:
   - Fever or chills with no other external urinary source noted.
   - Flank pain, suprapubic pain, tenderness, frequency, or urgency

- Worsening of mental or functional status
- Changes in urine character (e.g., new bloody urine, foul odor, increased sediment) and urinalysis or culture is not done
2. One of the following two signs or symptoms:
   - Fever or chills
   - Flank pain or suprapubic pain or tenderness

And both bacteriuria (determined by a positive urine culture for a potential pathogen or a positive nitrite assay by dipstick) and pyuria (determined by 10 or more white blood cells per high-power field on urinalysis or positive leukocyte esterase assay by dipstick).

Note: Asymptomatic UTIs are not included in these definitions.

Respiratory Tract Infections

Influenza-Like Illness (ILI). An ILI must meet both of the following criteria:

1. Fever
2. Presence of three of the following six signs or symptoms:
   - Chills
   - New headache or eye pain
   - Myalgia
   - Malaise or loss of appetite
   - Sore throat
   - New or increased cough

Note: This diagnosis will usually be made during influenza season: October through March, except in an influenza pandemic.
Note: During influenza season, if criteria for ILI and upper or lower respiratory tract infection are met at the same time, the infection should be recorded only as an ILI.

Lower Respiratory Infections (i.e., Bronchitis, Pneumonia). The patient has not had a chest film or the chest film did not confirm pneumonia and three of the following seven signs or symptoms are present:

1. New or increased cough
2. New or increased sputum production
3. New or increased purulence of sputum
4. Fever

5. Pleuritic chest pain
6. New or increased physical finding on chest examination
   - Rales
   - Rhonchi
   - Bronchial breathing
7. Change in status or breathing difficulty.
   - New or increased shortness of breath
   - Respiratory rate >25 per minute
   - Worsening mental or functional status

Note: Noninfectious causes, such as congestive heart failure, should be ruled out.

Note: If the patient has a chest X-ray interpreted as pneumonia, probable pneumonia or the presence of an infiltrate, and meets the above criteria for lower respiratory infections, it is counted as pneumonia.

Bloodstream Infections

Primary Bloodstream Infection. Primary bloodstream infection includes laboratory-confirmed bloodstream infection and clinical sepsis. A positive blood culture alone may be used to define bacteremia.

Laboratory-Confirmed Bloodstream Infection. Laboratory-confirmed bloodstream infection must meet one of the following three criteria:

1. Patient has a recognized pathogen cultured from one or more blood cultures *and* organism cultured from blood is not related to an infection at another site.
2. Patient has at least *one* of the following three signs or symptoms:
   - Fever
   - Chills
   - Hypotension

   And signs and symptoms and positive laboratory results that are not related to an infection at another site.

   And common skin contaminants (e.g., diphtheroids, *Bacillus* spp., *Propionibacterium* spp., coagulase-negative staphylococci, or micrococci) cultured from two or more blood cultures drawn on separate occasions.

3. Patient under one year of age has at least one of the following four signs or symptoms:
   - Fever
   - Hypothermia
   - Apnea
   - Bradycardia

   And signs and symptoms and positive laboratory results are not related to an infection at another site.

   And common skin contaminants (e.g., diphtheroids, *Bacillus* spp., *Propionibacterium* spp., coagulase-negative staphylococci, or micrococci) cultured from two or more blood cultures drawn on separate occasions.

Note: When an organism that is isolated from a blood culture is compatible with a related infection at another site, the bloodstream infection is classified as a secondary bloodstream infection

Note: Infections related to intravascular access devices are classified as primary, even if localized signs of infection are present at the access site.

Clinical Sepsis. Clinical sepsis must have at least one of the following clinical signs with no other recognized cause:

1. Fever
2. Hypotension (systolic pressure <90 mm Hg)
3. Oliguria (<20 mL/hr)
4. Hypothermia
5. Apnea
6. Bradycardia

   And blood culture is not done or no organisms detected in blood, and no apparent infection at another site.

   And physician institutes treatment for sepsis.

   And hospital admission for clinical sepsis or death due to clinical sepsis.

Intravenous Catheter Site Infection

Soft Tissue Infections. Cellulitis, soft tissue, nonsurgical wound, decubitus ulcer, foreign body site (e.g., gastrostomy, jejunostomy, tracheostomy), and around foreign body (e.g., PEGs, drains, catheters) infections must meet at least one of the following two criteria:

1. Purulent drainage at the wound, skin, or soft tissue site
2. Four or more of the following six signs or symptoms with no other recognized cause:
   - Fever or worsening mental or functional status
   - Pain or tenderness at the affected site
   - Localized swelling at the affected site
   - Redness at the affected site
   - Heat at the affected site
   - Serous discharge at the affected site

Skin Infections

Fungal Skin Infection. A fungal skin infection must meet both maculopapular rash and either physician diagnosis or laboratory confirmation must be present.

Herpes Simplex or Zoster Infection. A herpes simplex or zoster infection must meet both a vesicular rash and either physician diagnosis or laboratory confirmation must be present.

Surgical Site Infections (SSI). An SSI occurring within 30 days from the date of surgery is considered a HAI SSI. Infection related to a surgically implanted, nonhuman device is counted as an HAI SSI for up to 1 year from the date of surgery. An SSI meeting these criteria is reported to the facility where the surgery was performed, if information is available. Therefore, SSI definitions are included in the surveillance program for the home health and hospice care agency to assist in identifying the SSI before reporting their findings back to the facility where the surgical procedure was performed.

An SSI must meet both the following criteria:

1. Infection occurs within 30 days after the operative procedure if no implant is left in place or within one year if implant is in place and the infection appears to be related to the operative procedure
2. Two of the following seven signs or symptoms:
   - Purulent drainage from the incision or drain
   - Pain or tenderness

- Localized swelling and redness
- Heat
- Spontaneous dehiscence of the incision
- Fever

Note: SSIs should be considered HAIs and reported to the facility where the surgery was performed.

Eye, Ear, Nose, and Mouth Infections

Conjunctivitis. Infective conjunctivitis must meet one of the following two criteria:

1. Pus from one or both eyes
2. Redness with or without itching or pain

Note: Both trauma and allergies must be ruled out.

Ear Infection. An ear infection must meet one of the following two criteria:

1. Physician diagnosis
2. New purulent drainage fluid in the middle ear accompanied by ear pain or tympanic redness

Sinusitis. Sinusitis must meet at least one of the following three criteria:

1. Physician diagnosis
2. Organisms cultured from purulent material from the sinus cavity
3. One of the following four signs or symptoms with no other recognized cause:
   - Fever
   - Pain or tenderness over the involved sinus
   - Headache
   - Purulent exudates or nasal obstruction

Oral Infection. Oral infections must be physician diagnosed.

Note: Oral thrush is the presence of white patches in the oral cavity.

Gastrointestinal Infections

Gastroenteritis. Gastroenteritis must meet one of the following five criteria:

1. Two or more loose watery stools in 24 hours above what is normal for the patient
2. Two or more vomiting episodes in 24 hours
3. Vomiting
4. Abdominal pain or tenderness
5. Diarrhea

Note: Noninfectious causes, such as tube feeding or medication side effects, must be ruled out.

Clostridium difficile–Associated Diarrhea. Clostridium difficile-associated diarrhea meets all of the following three criteria:

1. Two or more loose watery stools in 24 hours above what is normal for the patient
2. A positive assay for *Clostridium difficile* toxin
3. Both a stool culture positive for a gastrointestinal pathogen *and* any of the following four signs or symptoms:
   a. Nausea
   b. Vomiting
   c. Abdominal cramping or pain
   d. Fever

Note: Report suspected Clostridium difficile-associated diarrhea to the healthcare facility from which the patient was discharged.

Reporting Patient Infection

All patient infections occurring up to 30 days after discharge are to be reported to the attending physician and the medical facility from which the patient was discharged. This is in keeping with the definition of an HAI.

Documentation of signs and symptoms suggestive of infection, reporting, and medical follow-up need to be documented (table 6–24). Table 6–25 on page 62 is a sample for documentation and reporting.

Table 6-24. Reporting infectious and communicable diseases[23]

Procedure	Rationale/Action
All HAIs occurring post discharge must be reported.	This is requirement under the rules set forth by CMS.
All HAIs must be reported to the medical facility from which the patient was discharged and the patients attending physician must also be notified.	Tracking of HAIs is a CMS requirement.
The Public Health Service has defined diseases that are required to be reported by law.	This assists the CDC in tracking on a national level.
Refer to state list of reportable diseases.	Disease listing may vary from state to state. Obtain a copy from your health department.
If a reportable disease is identified and diagnosed, it is to be reported to the local Public Health Department.	A fine can be imposed for a failure to report.
Notify the patient's case manager.	
Document in patient's record and report file.	

Administration of Vaccines and Immunizations

Old diseases such as measles, mumps and rubella, chickenpox, and pertussis (whooping cough) have returned. Some CP and MIH groups are offering vaccine and immunization services to persons in the community as part of increasing health and welfare. This is a great service, especially in rural and underserved population areas.

Since the administration of vaccines and immunizations are not generally in the scope of practice, this issue must be investigated before offering these services. For example, in the state of Virginia, the scope of paramedic practice was expanded to include the administration of vaccines and immunizations. All the appropriate medications were added to the drug formulary. This enables paramedics in the state to not only offer services to the public, but also to conduct programs in-house and eliminate the cost of contracting these services for the department.

Once the scope of practice is revised, there is a need to review injection technique, skin prep education regarding possible side effects, allergy issues, and possible contraindications.

Table 6-25. CP and MIH infection control log

Monthly Report: _____
Postdischarge: _____

Patient	CP/MIH Admit Date	Infection Onset Date	Site	Infection Related DX	Culture Yes/ Date	Culture No	X-Ray Date	Organism	Antibiotic	Recultured Date	Date Resolved

Total Number of Infections				Healthcare Associated Infections	
Skin:		UTI/Catheter-associated UTI:		Upper Respiratory:		Gastrointestinal:		Date reported to Infection Control/Performance Improvement Committee:	_/_/_
Eye:		Urinary Tract:		Lower Respiratory:		Other, Specify:			

The following information is to assist in meeting the infection control aspects of this topic (tables 6–26 and 6–27).

Table 6–26. Skin preparation for vaccine injection in home care[25]

Procedure	Rationale/Action*
Wash hands *with* soap and warm water.	
If not available, use alcohol gel or foam.	Basic infection prevention.
Gloves are not necessary to give an injection.	Per OSHA Bloodborne Pathogens Regulation Compliance Directive CPL 02-02-069[a] and CDC guidelines.
Observe skin at injection site.	*Avoid* giving injections if skin is compromised by local infection or other skin conditions: weeping, dermatitis, skin lesions, or cuts.
Wipe the area from the center of the injection site working in a circular motion outward.	Do *not* go back to the center of the site.
Allow to dry.	

*Enforcement Procedures for the Occupational Exposure to Bloodborne Pathogens, CPL 02-02-069 (2001).

Table 6–27. Skin preparation for different types of injection[24]

	Skin Preparation and Disinfection	
Type of Injection	Soap and Water	60–70% Alcohol (isopropyl alcohol or ethanol)
Intradermal	Yes	No
Subcutaneous	Yes	No
Intramuscular		
• Immunization	Yes	No*
• Therapeutic	Yes	Yes
Venous Access	No	Yes

Do *not* use alcohol skin disinfection for administration of vaccinations.

*This is an unresolved issue, because there is insufficient evidence on the need to disinfect the skin with alcohol before an intramuscular injection to change the 2003 World Health Organization recommendation; further studies are warranted.

Table 6–28. Guide to Vaccine Contraindications from the CDC[26]

Vaccine	Contraindications	Precautions
Influenza, inactivated (IIV) Influenza, recombinant	Severe allergic reaction (e.g., anaphylaxis) after a previous dose or to a vaccine component	Moderate or severe acute illness with or without fever
		History of Guillain-Barré Syndrome within 6 weeks of previous influenza vaccination
		For IIV vaccine only: Egg allergy other than hives (e.g., angioedema, respiratory distress, lightheadedness, or recurrent emesis); or required epinephrine or another emergency medical intervention (IIV may be administered in an inpatient or outpatient medical setting under the supervision of a healthcare provider who is able to recognize and manage severe allergic conditions)
Tetanus, diphtheria, pertussis Tetanus, diphtheria	Severe allergic reaction (e.g., anaphylaxis) after a previous dose or to a vaccine component	Moderate or severe acute illness with or without fever
	For pertussis-containing vaccines: encephalopathy (e.g., coma, decreased level of consciousness, or prolonged seizures) not attributable to another identifiable cause within 7 days of administration of a previous dose of a vaccine containing tetanus or diphtheria toxoid or acellular pertussis.	Guillain-Barré Syndrome within 6 weeks after a previous dose of tetanus toxoid-containing vaccine
		History of Arthus-type hypersensitivity reactions after a previous dose of tetanus or diphtheria toxoid-containing vaccine (including MenACWY); defer vaccination until at least 10 years have elapsed since the last tetanus toxoid-containing vaccine.
		For pertussis-containing vaccines: progressive or unstable neurologic disorder, uncontrolled seizures, or progressive encephalopathy until a treatment regimen has been established and the condition has stabilized
Varicella	Severe allergic reaction (e.g., anaphylaxis) after a previous dose or to a vaccine component	Moderate or severe acute illness with or without fever
	Severe immunodeficiency (e.g., hematologic and solid tumors, chemotherapy, congenital immunodeficiency, or long-term immunosuppressive therapy), or persons with human immunodeficiency virus (HIV) infection who are severely immunocompromised.	Recent (within 11 months) receipt of antibody-containing blood product (specific interval depends on product)
		Receipt of specific antivirals (i.e., acyclovir, famciclovir, or valacyclovir) 24 hours before vaccination; avoid use of these antiviral drugs for 14 days after vaccination
	Pregnancy	

Vaccine	Contraindications	Precautions
Human papillomavirus	Severe allergic reaction (e.g., anaphylaxis) after a previous dose or to a vaccine component	Moderate or severe acute illness with or without fever
		Pregnancy
Herpes zoster	Severe allergic reaction (e.g., anaphylaxis) to a vaccine component	Moderate or severe acute illness with or without fever
	Severe immunodeficiency (e.g., from hematologic and solid tumors, receipt of chemotherapy, or long-term immunosuppressive therapy), or persons with HIV infection who are severely immunocompromised.	Receipt of specific antivirals (i.e., acyclovir, famciclovir, or valacyclovir) 24 hours before vaccination; avoid use of these antiviral drugs for 14 days after vaccination
	Pregnancy	
Measles, mumps, rubella	Severe allergic reaction (e.g., anaphylaxis) after a previous dose or to a vaccine component	Moderate or severe acute illness with or without fever
	Severe immunodeficiency (e.g., hematologic and solid tumors, chemotherapy, congenital immunodeficiency, or long-term immunosuppressive therapy), or persons with HIV infection who are severely immunocompromised.	Recent (within 11 months) receipt of antibody-containing blood product (specific interval depends on product)
		History of thrombocytopenia or thrombocytopenic purpura
		Need for tuberculin skin testing[9]
	Pregnancy	
Pneumococcal: conjugate (PCV13), polysaccharide	Severe allergic reaction (e.g., anaphylaxis) after a previous dose or to a vaccine component (including, for PCV13, to any vaccine containing diphtheria toxoid-containing vaccine	Moderate or severe acute illness with or without fever
Hepatitis A	Severe allergic reaction (e.g., anaphylaxis) after a previous dose or to a vaccine component	Moderate or severe acute illness with or without fever
Hepatitis B	Severe allergic reaction (e.g., anaphylaxis) after a previous dose or to a vaccine component	Moderate or severe acute illness with or without fever
	Hypersensitivity to yeast	
Meningococcal: conjugate (MenACWY), serogroup B (MemB)*	Severe allergic reaction (e.g., anaphylaxis) after a previous dose or to a vaccine component	Moderate or severe acute illness with or without fever
Haemophilus influenzae type B	Severe allergic reaction (e.g., anaphylaxis) after a previous dose or to a vaccine component	Moderate or severe acute illness with or without fever

*There is now a vaccine that includes MenB, therefore 5 types of meningococcal are covered in one vaccine:
- Penbraya is indicated for active immunization to prevent invasive disease caused by *Neisseria meningitidis* serogroups A, B, C, W, and Y. Penbraya is approved for use in individuals 10 through 25 years of age.
- Trumenba is indicated for active immunization to prevent invasive disease caused by *Neisseria meningitidis* serogroup B. Trumenba is approved for use in individuals 10 through 25 years of age.

Source. "Use of Pfizer Pentavalent Meningococcal Vaccine Among Persons Aged >10 Years: Recommendations for the Advisory Committee on Immunization Practices-United States, 2023," *Morbidity and Mortality Weekly Report 73*, no.15 (2024): 345–50.

Screening Checklist for Contraindications to Vaccines for Adults

YOUR NAME _____

DATE OF BIRTH ___/___/___
               month day year

For patients: The following questions will help us determine which vaccines you may be given today. If you answer "yes" to any question, it does not necessarily mean you should not be vaccinated. It just means we need to ask you more questions. If a question is not clear, please ask your healthcare provider to explain it.

	yes	no	don't know
1. Are you sick today?	☐	☐	☐
2. Do you have allergies to medications, food, a vaccine component, or latex?	☐	☐	☐
3. Have you ever had a serious reaction after receiving a vaccine?	☐	☐	☐
4. Do you have any of the following: a long-term health problem with heart, lung, kidney, or metabolic disease (e.g., diabetes), asthma, a blood disorder, no spleen, a cochlear implant, or a spinal fluid leak? Are you on long-term aspirin therapy?	☐	☐	☐
5. Do you have cancer, leukemia, HIV/AIDS, or any other immune system problem?	☐	☐	☐
6. Do you have a parent, brother, or sister with an immune system problem?	☐	☐	☐
7. In the past 6 months, have you taken medications that affect your immune system, such as prednisone, other steroids, or anticancer drugs; drugs for the treatment of rheumatoid arthritis, Crohn's disease, or psoriasis; or have you had radiation treatments?	☐	☐	☐
8. Have you had a seizure or a brain or other nervous system problem?	☐	☐	☐
9. Have you ever been diagnosed with a heart condition (myocarditis or pericarditis) or have you had Multisystem Inflammatory Syndrome (MIS-A or MIS-C) after an infection with the virus that causes COVID-19?	☐	☐	☐
10. In the past year, have you received immune (gamma) globulin, blood/blood products, or an antiviral drug?	☐	☐	☐
11. Are you pregnant?	☐	☐	☐
12. Have you received any vaccinations in the past 4 weeks?	☐	☐	☐
13. Have you ever felt dizzy or faint before, during, or after a shot?	☐	☐	☐
14. Are you anxious about getting a shot today?	☐	☐	☐

FORM COMPLETED BY _____ DATE _____

FORM REVIEWED BY _____ DATE _____

Did you bring your immunization record card with you?   yes ☐   no ☐

It is important to have a personal record of your vaccinations. If you don't have a personal record, ask your healthcare provider to give you one. Keep this record in a safe place and bring it with you every time you seek medical care. Make sure your healthcare provider records all your vaccinations on it.

Immunize.org

FOR PROFESSIONALS www.immunize.org / FOR THE PUBLIC www.vaccineinformation.org

www.immunize.org/catg.d/p4065.pdf
Item #P4065 (12/10/2024)

Figure 6–8. Screening checklist for contraindications to vaccines for adults[27]

Information for Healthcare Professionals about the Screening Checklist for Contraindications to Vaccines for Adults

Are you interested in knowing why we included a certain question on the screening checklist? If so, read the information below. If you want to find out even more, consult the references listed at the end.

1. Are you sick today? *[all vaccines]*

There is no evidence that acute illness reduces vaccine efficacy or increases vaccine adverse events.[1] However, as a precaution with moderate or severe acute illness, all vaccines should be delayed until the illness has improved. Mild illnesses (such as upper respiratory infections or diarrhea) are NOT contraindications to vaccination. Do not withhold vaccination if a person is taking antibiotics.

2. Do you have allergies to medications, food, a vaccine component, or latex? *[all vaccines]*

An anaphylactic reaction to latex is a contraindication to vaccines that contain latex as a component or as part of the packaging (e.g., vial stoppers, prefilled syringe plungers, prefilled syringe caps). If a person has anaphylaxis after eating gelatin, do not administer vaccines containing gelatin. A local reaction to a prior vaccine dose or vaccine component, including latex, is not a contraindication to a subsequent dose or vaccine containing that component. For information on vaccines supplied in vials or syringes containing latex, see reference 2; for an extensive list of vaccine components, see reference 3.

People with egg allergy of any severity can receive any IIV, RIV, or LAIV that is otherwise appropriate for the patient's age and health status. The safety of LAIV in egg allergic people has not been established. For people with a history of severe allergic reaction to egg involving any symptom other than hives (e.g., angioedema, respiratory distress), or who required epinephrine or another emergency medical intervention, the vaccine should be administered in a medical setting, such as a clinic, health department, or physician office. Vaccine administration should be supervised by a healthcare provider who is able to recognize and manage severe allergic conditions.[4]

3. Have you ever had a serious reaction after receiving a vaccination? *[all vaccines]*

History of anaphylactic reaction (see question 2) to a previous dose of vaccine or vaccine component is a contraindication for subsequent doses.[1] Under normal circumstances, vaccines are deferred when a precaution is present. However, situations may arise when the benefit outweighs the risk (e.g., during a community pertussis outbreak).

4. Do you have a long-term health problem with heart, lung, kidney, or metabolic disease (e.g., diabetes), asthma, a blood disorder, no spleen, component component deficiency, a cochlear implant, or a spinal fluid leak? Are you on long term aspirin therapy? *[MMR, VAR, LAIV]*

A history of thrombocytopenia or thrombocytopenic purpura is a precaution to MMR vaccine. LAIV is not recommended for people with anatomic or functional asplenia, complement component deficiency, a cochlear implant, or CSF leak.[5] These conditions, including asthma in adults, should be considered precautions for the use of LAIV. Aspirin use is a precaution to VAR.

5. Do you, or does a close family member, have cancer, leukemia, HIV/AIDS, or any other immune system problem? *[LAIV, MMR, VAR, ZVL]*

Live virus vaccines (e.g., LAIV, measles-mumps-rubella [MMR], varicella [VAR], zoster vaccine live [ZVL]) are usually contraindicated in immunocompromised people. However, there are exceptions. For example, MMR vaccine is recommended and varicella vaccine should be considered for adults with CD4+ T-lymphocyte counts of greater than or equal to 200 cells/μL. Immunosuppressed people should not receive LAIV. For details, consult the ACIP recommendations.[4,6,7]

6. In the past 3 months, have you taken medications that affect your immune system, such as cortisone, prednisone, other steroids, or anticancer drugs; drugs for the treatment of rheumatoid arthritis, Crohn's disease, or psoriasis; or have you had radiation treatments? *[LAIV, MMR, VAR, ZVL]*

Live virus vaccines (e.g., LAIV, MMR, VAR, ZVL) should be postponed until after chemotherapy or long-term high-dose steroid therapy has ended. For details and length of time to postpone, consult the ACIP statement.[1,6] Some immune mediator and immune modulator drugs (especially the anti-tumor necrosis factor agents adalimumab, infliximab, etanercept, golimumab, and certolizumab pegol) may be immunosuppressive. A comprehensive list of immunosuppressive immune modulators is available in CDC Health Information for International Travel (the "Yellow Book") available at wwwnc.cdc.gov/travel/yellowbook/2018/advising-travelers-with-specific-needs/immunocompromised-travelers The use of live vaccines should be avoided in persons taking these drugs (see www.cdc.gov/vaccines/hcp/acip-recs/general-recs/contraindications.html). To find specific vaccination schedules for stem cell transplant (bone marrow transplant) patients, see reference 7. LAIV can be given only to healthy non-pregnant people ages 2 through 49 years.

7. Have you had a seizure or a brain or other nervous system problem? *[influenza, Td/Tdap]*

Tdap is contraindicated in people who have a history of encephalopathy within 7 days following DTP/DTaP. An unstable progressive neurologic problem is a precaution to the use of Tdap. For people with stable neurologic disorders (including seizures) unrelated to vaccination, or for people with a family history of seizure, vaccinate as usual. A history of Guillain-Barré syndrome (GBS) is a consideration with the following: 1) Td/Tdap: if GBS has occurred within 6 weeks of a tetanus-toxoid vaccine and decision is made to continue vaccination, give Tdap instead of Td if no history of prior Tdap; 2) Influenza vaccine (IIV/LAIV): if GBS has occurred within 6 weeks of a prior influenza vaccine, vaccinate with IIV if at increased risk for severe influenza complications.

8. During the past year, have you received a transfusion of blood or blood products, or been given immune (gamma) globulin or an antiviral drug? *[MMR, VAR]*

Certain live virus vaccines (e.g., MMR, VAR) may need to be deferred, depending on several variables. Consult the most current ACIP recommendations for current information on intervals between antiviral drugs, immune globulin or blood product administration and live virus vaccines.[1]

9. For women: Are you pregnant or is there a chance you could become pregnant during the next month? *[HPV, IPV, MMR, LAIV, VAR, ZVL]*

Live virus vaccines (e.g., MMR, VAR, ZVL, LAIV) are contraindicated one month before and during pregnancy because of the theoretical risk of virus transmission to the fetus. Sexually active women in their childbearing years who receive live virus vaccines should be instructed to avoid pregnancy for one month following receipt of the vaccine. On theoretical grounds, inactivated poliovirus vaccine should not be given during pregnancy; however, it may be given if risk of exposure is imminent and immediate protection is needed (e.g., travel to endemic areas). Inactivated influenza vaccine and Tdap are both recommended during pregnancy. Both vaccines may be given at any time during pregnancy but the preferred time for Tdap administration is at 27–36 weeks' gestation. HPV vaccine is not recommended during pregnancy.[1,4,6,8,9,10]

10. Have you received any vaccinations in the past 4 weeks? *[LAIV, MMR, VAR, yellow fever, ZVL]*

People who were given either LAIV or an injectable live virus vaccine (e.g., MMR, VAR, ZVL, yellow fever) should wait 28 days before receiving another vaccination of this type (30 days for yellow fever). Inactivated vaccines may be given at any spacing interval if they are not administered simultaneously.

REFERENCES

1. CDC. General best practice guidelines for immunization. Best Practices Guidance of the Advisory Committee on Immunization Practices (ACIP) at www.cdc.gov/vaccines/hcp/acip-recs/general-recs/index.html.
2. Latex in Vaccine Packaging: www.cdc.gov/vaccines/pubs/pinkbook/downloads/appendices/B/latex-table.pdf.
3. Table of Vaccine Components: www.cdc.gov/vaccines/pubs/pinkbook/downloads/appendices/B/excipient-table-2.pdf.
4. CDC. Prevention and control of seasonal influenza with vaccines: Recommendations of the Advisory Committee on Immunization Practices – United States, . . . Access links to current ACIP recommendations at www.cdc.gov/vaccines/hcp/acip-recs/vacc-specific/flu.html
5. CDC. Recommended Adult Immunization Schedule for Ages 19 Years or older at https://www.cdc.gov/vaccines/schedules/downloads/adult/adult-combined-schedule.pdf
6. CDC. Measles, mumps, and rubella – vaccine use and strategies for elimination of measles, rubella, and congenital rubella syndrome and control of mumps. *MMWR* 1998; 47 (RR-8).
7. CDC. Prevention of varicella: Recommendations of the Advisory Committee on Immunization Practices. *MMWR* 2007; 56 (RR-4).
8. Tomblyn M, Einsele H, et al. Guidelines for preventing infectious complications among hematopoietic stem cell transplant recipients: a global perspective. Biol Blood Marrow Transplant 15:1143–1238; 2009 at www.cdc.gov/vaccines/pubs/hemato-cell-transplts.htm.
9. CDC. Notice to readers: Revised ACIP recommendation for avoiding pregnancy after receiving a rubella-containing vaccine. *MMWR* 2001; 50 (49).
10. CDC. Updated recommendations for use of tetanus toxoid, reduced diphtheria toxoid, and acellular pertussis vaccine (Tdap) in pregnant women: Recommendations of the ACIP. *MMWR* 2012; 62 (7):131–4.

Immunization Action Coalition • Saint Paul, Minnesota • 651-647-9009 • www.immunize.org • www.vaccineinformation.org

www.immunize.org/catg.d/p4065.pdf • Item #P4065 – page 2 (4/19)

Figure 6–9. Information for healthcare professionals about the screening checklist for contraindications to vaccines for adults[28]

Compliance Monitoring

Compliance monitoring is an OSHA requirement. Compliance monitoring is designed to evaluate the healthcare provider's compliance with policies and procedures.

Rationale
- Ensuring that your program is working
- Ensure staff knows their responsibilities
- Obtain information for annual performance appraisals
- Document for medical facility inquiries

This is clearly stated in the OSH Act of 1970 in Section 5 Duties (b) which states

> "Each employee shall comply with occupational safety and health standards and all rules, regulations, and orders issued pursuant to the Act which are applicable to his own actions and conduct."[15]

How Should This Be Done and By Whom?
The gold standard for monitoring is direct observation. This scan should be performed by supervisors and the results reported to the department designated infection control officer.

How Often Should This Be Performed?
Frequency depends on the results of the initial observations. If there is a good percentage for compliance on a procedure, then annual monitoring may be appropriate. If the compliance percentage is in the 70%–80% range, then quarterly monitoring would be indicated. However, if compliance is below the 70% range, then monthly monitoring should be started along with sharing the results with the training officer to be addressed in annual update training.

Medical facilities are now looking at EMS performance as a possible source for patient infections. Compliance monitories will be of assistance in demonstrating that policies and procedures for infection control are being followed.

Why Is This Important?
It is important to demonstrate how care providers are following the policies and procedures established for home care and adopted by the department for risk and liability reduction.

One study conducted and presented in 2014 at an international conference in France examined data on 5,954 patients from 179 volunteer home care settings. Half of the patients had received home care for at least 35 days; only 2.3% received home care for less than 2 days. Of the 420 HAIs reported in 403 patients, 35.5% were acquired in the home.

Overall, 6.8% of patients developed at least one active HAI, and 2.5% developed at least one infection from home care. The most frequently isolated microorganism was Staphylococcus aureus, at 20.7%, and 28.1% of those cases were methicillin-resistant. The primary infections were in the urinary tract (43.0%) and the respiratory tract.

At a time when medical facilities are not receiving reimbursement for HAIs and are being penalized for increased readmissions, it is important to be able to document compliance with established policies and procedures.

Definition of Terms

Bloodborne pathogens are pathogenic microorganisms that are present in human blood and can cause disease in humans. These pathogens include, but are not limited to, the hepatitis B virus, the hepatitis C virus, and the human immunodeficiency virus.

Contaminated means the presence or the reasonably anticipated presence of blood or other potentially infectious materials on an item or surface.

Contaminated sharps are any contaminated objects that can penetrate the skin including, but not limited to, needles, scalpels, broken glass, and broken capillary tubes.

Decontamination is using physical or chemical means to remove, inactivate, or destroy bloodborne pathogens on a surface or item to the point where they are no longer capable of transmitting infectious particles and the surface or item is rendered safe for handling, use, or disposal.

Engineering controls are controls that isolate or remove the bloodborne pathogens hazard from the workplace. Examples include sharps disposal containers, self-sheathing needles, and safer medical devices like sharps with engineered sharps injury protections and needleless systems.

Healthcare-associated infection (HAI) is either an infection that occurs two days after admission and is unrelated to the admission diagnosis, or an infection that occurs 30 days after discharge.

Exposure incidents mean that as a result of an employee's performance duties, blood or other potentially infectious materials have been in contact with the parenteral area, broken skin, an eye, mouth, or another mucous membrane.

Home care–associated infections are infections that develop in the home care situation.

Occupational exposure means reasonably anticipated skin, eye, mucous membrane, or parenteral contact with blood or other potentially infectious materials that may result from the performance of an employee's duties.

Other potentially infectious materials include the following human body fluids:

- Semen and vaginal secretions (only at risk through sexual contact)
- Cerebrospinal, synovial, pleural, pericardial, peritoneal, and amniotic fluid
- Saliva in dental procedures
- Any body fluid that is visibly contaminated with blood
- All body fluids in situations where it is difficult or impossible to differentiate between body fluids

Personal protective equipment (PPE) is specialized clothing or equipment worn by an employee for protection against a hazard. General work clothes (e.g., uniforms, pants, shirts, or blouses) not intended to function as protection against a hazard are not considered to be personal protective equipment.

Sharps with engineered sharps injury protections are a nonneedle sharp or a needle device used for withdrawing body fluids, accessing a vein or artery, or administering medications or other fluids that has a built-in safety feature or mechanism that effectively reduces the risk of an exposure incident.

Source individuals (patients) are any individuals, living or dead, whose blood or other potentially infectious materials may be a source of occupational exposure to the employee. Examples include, but are not limited to, hospital and clinic patients, clients in institutions for the developmentally disabled, trauma victims, clients of drug and alcohol treatment facilities, residents of hospices and nursing homes, human remains, and individuals who donate or sell blood or blood components.

Standard precaution is an approach to infection control. According to the concept of Universal Standard Precautions, all human blood and certain human body fluids (except sweat) are treated as if known to be infectious for human immunodeficiency virus, hepatitis B virus, hepatitis C virus, and other blood-borne pathogens.

Regulated waste includes the following:

- Liquid or semiliquid blood or other potentially infectious materials
- Contaminated items that would release blood or other potentially infectious materials in a liquid or semiliquid state if compressed
- Items that are caked with dried blood or other potentially infectious materials and are capable of releasing these materials during handling
- Contaminated sharps
- Pathological and microbiological wastes containing blood or other potentially infectious materials

Each state has specific regulations to reference. Table 6–29 can be used for monitoring compliance.

OSHA enforces the medical waste regulations for each state. These are not in this book.

Table 6-29. CP or MIH compliance quality monitor

Date:

Criteria	Compliance YES	Compliance NO	Observations/Notes	% Complaint
General home area is clean				
Patient education materials are available				
Patient health history was obtained				
Bathrooms are clean				
Hand-washing solutions are available				
Hand-washing solutions are filled				
Proper handwashing is observed				
Personal protective attire is readily available				
Gloves were used in accordance with policy				
Gloves were changed in accordance with policy				
Masks were used per policy				
Protective eyewear was used in accordance with policy				
Uniforms/aprons/cover gowns were used in accordance with policy				
Staff compliant in proper use of personal protective equipment				
• Donning of PPE				
• Doffing of PPE				
Action/Follow up:			Date for next review:	

Table 6-29. CP or MIH compliance quality monitor (*continued*)

Date:				
Criteria	Compliance YES	Compliance NO	Observations/Notes	% Complaint
Aseptic technique was practiced during the procedure				
Heavy duty gloves were used for cleaning surfaces and instruments				
Surface cleaning agent is dated and mixed according to recommendations				
Multidose vials are properly dated and stored				
Excess medications disposed of according to local regulations				
Separate refrigerator for food and medications				
Action/Follow up:		Date for next review:		

Table 6–29. CP or MIH compliance quality monitor (continued)

Date:				
Criteria	Compliance YES	Compliance NO	Observations/Notes	% Complaint
Patient record is properly maintained				
Patient record notes each visit and care rendered				
Patient signed permission for testing if an exposure occurred				
Foley catheter is properly positioned				
IV site observed for infection and infiltration				
Irrigation solutions are dated				
Staff is aware of procedure for reporting exposures				
Staff is aware or procedure for reporting communicable diseases				
Staff is aware of procedure for disposal of unused medications				
Staff using proper site prep solutions				
Sharps are disposed of in proper containers of unused medications				
Heavy duty dishwashing gloves are used for cleaning				
Action/Follow Up:			Date for Next Review:	

Notes

1. Brenda Luther et al., "Discharge Processes: What Evidence Tells Us Is Most Effective," *Orthopaedic Nursing* 38, no. 5 (2019): 328–33.
2. Luther et al., "Discharge Processes," 328–33.
3. "Home Health Care vs. Hospital Care," Healthstream, April 1, 2021, https://www.healthstream.com/resource/blog/home-health-care-vs.-hospital-care.
4. Luther et al., "Discharge Processes," 328–33.
5. Henil Patel and Daniel West, Jr., "Hospital at Home: An Evolving Model for Comprehensive Healthcare," *Global Journal of Quality and Safety in Healthcare* 4, no. 4 (2021): 141–46, https://doi.org/10.36401/JQSH-21-4.
6. Luther et al., "Discharge Processes," 328–33.
7. Jingjing Shang et al., "Infection in Home Healthcare: Results from National Outcome and Assessment Information Set Data," *American Journal of Infection Control* 5, vol. 43 (2015): 454–59.
8. APIC Home Care Membership Section, "APIC-HICPAC Surveillance Definitions for Home Health Care and Home Hospice Infections," Association for Professionals in Infection Control and Epidemiology, February 2008.
9. Naomi O'Grady et al., "Guidelines for the Prevention of Intravascular Catheter-related Infections," *Clinical Infectious Diseases* 9, vol. 52 (2011): 1087–99.
10. Sailaritta Vuorisalo et al., "Treatment of Diabetic Foot Ulcers," *Journal of Cardiovascular Surgery (Torino)* 3, vol. 50 (2009): 275–91.
11. William Rutala et al., *Guidelines for Sterilization and Disinfection* (Centers for Disease Control & Prevention, 2008); OSHA Regulation 1910.1036, Hand Protection–Gloves.
12. "Summary of Recommendations," in *Guideline for Prevention of Catheter-Associated Urinary Tract Infections* (Centers for Disease Control and Prevention, 2009).
13. Kevin Lewis and Jeffrey Pay, "Wound Irrigation," in *StatPearls* (2023).
14. "Disposal of Unused Medicines," Food and Drug Administration, https://www.fda.gov/drugs/safe-disposal-medicines/disposal-unused-medicines-what-you-should-know
15. "Duties," Occupational Safety and Health Act of 1970, 29 U.S.C. § 654.
16. Emily Rhinehart, "Infection Control in Home Care."
17. *Caring for Your Feet*, West Virginia Medical Institute.
18. Ron Rajecki, "Reducing Ostomy Infection Risk," I Advance Senior Care, 2014, https://www.iadvanceseniorcare.com/reducing-ostomy-infection-risk/.
19. "Tracheostomy Care," Cleveland Clinic, https://health.clevelandclinic.org/trach-care.
20. Michael Edmonds, "Diabetic Foot Ulcers: Practical Treatment Recommendations," *Drugs 7*, no. 66 (2006): 913–29.
21. *Caring for Your Feet*, West Virginia Medical Institute.
22. "Safe Injection Practices and Your Health," Centers for Disease Control, 2024, https://www.cdc.gov/injection-safety/about/index.html.
23. "Healthcare Facility HAI Reporting Requirements to CMS via NHSN Current or Proposed Requirements," Centers for Disease Control and Prevention, 2022, https://bpb-us-w2.wpmucdn.com/u.osu.edu/dist/c/28860/files/2016/11/cms-reporting-requirements-1opk92x.pdf
24. *WHO Best Practices for Injections and Related Procedures Toolkit* (World Health Organization, 2010).

25. "Use of Pfizer Pentavalent Meningococcal Vaccine Among Persons Aged >10 Years: Recommendations for the Advisory Committee on Immunization Practices—United States, 2023," *Morbidity and Mortality Weekly Report 73*, no.15 (2024): 345–50.
26. "Contraindications and Precautions," Vaccines and Immunizations, Centers for Disease Control and Prevention, last updated July 25,2024, https://www.cdc.gov/vaccines/hcp/imz-best-practices/contraindications-precautions.html.
27. "Screening Checklist for Contraindications to Vaccines for Adults," Immunize.org, updated December 10, 2024, https://www.immunize.org/wp-content/uploads/catg.d/p4065.pdf.
28. "Information for Healthcare Professionals about the Screening Checklist for Contraindications to Vaccines for Adults," Immunize.org, updated December 10, 2024, https://www.immunize.org/wp-content/uploads/catg.d/p4065.pdf.

Index

A
ACA (Affordable Care Act) xi
acellular pertussis (Tdap) 5
Affordable Care Act (ACA) xi
airborne/droplet exposures 25
American Journal of Infection Control xii

B
bleach and general cleaning 49
bloodborne exposure
    defined 21
    human immunodeficiency virus (HIV) 1, 23
    sharps disposal 49
    testing 23–24
blood drawing 28
bloodstream infections (BSI)
    clinical sepsis (CSEP) 57
    primary 56
body fluids safe unless blood present 21–22
bronchitis 55
BSI. *See* bloodstream infections (BSI)

C
catheter-associated urinary tract infections (CAUTI) 44, 54
catheters
    healthcare-associated infections (HAIs) 42
    home care 43
    improper maintenance 42
    maintenance 42–44
    peripherally-inserted central catheters (PICCs) 42
    site infection 57
    transporting patients with 44
    urinary tract infection 44, 54
CDAD (clostridium difficile-associated diarrhea) 60
CDC. *See* Centers for Disease Control (CDC)
Center for Medicare and Medicaid Services (CMS) xi
    discharge instructions and xi
Centers for Disease Control (CDC) 5, 23, 27
    personal protective equipment guidelines 27
    work restriction guidelines 7–13
chickenpox 61
cleaning patient care equipment. *See also* general cleaning
    costs 31
    disinfection 31–32
Clinical Laboratory Improvement Amendment (CLIA). 23
clinical sepsis (CSEP) 57
Clostridium difficile-associated diarrhea (CDAD) 60
CMS. *See* Center for Medicare and Medicaid Services (CMS)
community paramedicine (CP) xii, 1, 22, 33
    exposure risks 22
compliance
    frequency 68
    handwashing 16
    monitoring 68
    terms 69
conjunctivitis 59

contact precautions 29–30
   high touch items 29, 49
COVID-19 pandemic xi
   work restrictions 13
CP. See community paramedicine (CP)
CSEP (clinical sepsis) 57

D

declination form 6
   work restrictions 7
designated infection control officer (DICO)
   creation 1
   exposure reporting to 23
   patient testing 23
   responsibilities 2
   vaccine record access 7
diabetic foot ulcers
   assessment 49
   care 46–49
   picking shoes 48
DICO. See designated infection control officer (DICO)
diphtheria 5
discharge
   documentation 36
   food security 33
   instructions xi
   mobility restrictions 36
   nursing staff 33
   patient understanding 36
   planners 33
   primary care physician contact 33
   summary 33, 36
diseases. See infections
disinfection improper 31
drawing blood 28
dressing change 38
droplet precautions 30
Duke University 31

E

ear infection 59
emergency care, prehospital 16, 22
emergency medical services (EMS) xi
   communication 38
   hospital to home care (HaH) role 36
   medical record maintenance 33, 36
   patient testing 23
   scope of practice 23
   surgical wound care 38
   vaccine requirements 5–6
emergency medical technician (EMT)
   scope of practice 22
EMS. See emergency medical services (EMS)
exposures. See also bloodborne exposure
   airborne/droplet exposures 25
   low-risk patient 24
   mobile-integrated healthcare (MIH) 22
   postexposure procedures 22
   reporting to DICO 23
   risks 22
eye, ear, nose, and mouth infections
   conjunctivitis 59
   ear infection 59
   oral infection 59
   sinusitis 59

F

FDA (Food & Drug Administration) 23
fingerstick pens disposal 49
Food & Drug Administration (FDA) 23
food security 33
fungal skin infection 58

G

gastroenteritis 60
general cleaning. See also cleaning patient care equipment
   bleach 49
   glucose-monitoring device 49
   high touch items 29, 49
   humidifiers 49
General Duty Clause 2, 6–8
gloves
   handwashing and 17
   nitrile and latex allergies and 17
   personal protective equipment 16
glucose-monitoring device general cleaning 49

H

HaH. See hospital to home care (HaH)
HAI. See healthcare-associated infections (HAIs)

handwashing 31
   compared to gloves 17
   compliance 16
   healthcare-associated infections (HAIs) 31
HCV (hepatitis C virus) 23
healthcare-associated infections (HAIs)
   catheters 42
   handwashing 31
   improper disinfection 31
   preventability 31
Healthcare Infection Control Practices Advisory Committee (HICPAC) 31
   CDC collaboration 31
hepatitis B 7, 23
hepatitis C virus (HCV) 23
herpes simplex 58
HICPAC. *See* Healthcare Infection Control Practices Advisory Committee (HICPAC)
hierarchy of safety controls. *See* safety controls
high-risk patients 24
high touch items 29, 49
HIV. *See* human immunodeficiency virus
home care environment xi
   catheters 43
   home evaluation 33
   infection assessment 52
   infections xii
   personal protective equipment (PPE) 27–28
   postexposure procedures 22
   safety checklist 35
home safety 34
hospital to home care (HaH)
   benefits 34
   emergency medical services role 36
   terminology 37
   training 34
human immunodeficiency virus (HIV) 1, 23
   rapid testing 23
humidifiers 49

I

ILI (influenza-like illness) 55
infections. *See also* eye, ear, nose, and mouth infections; multi-drug resistant infections; skin infections
   acellular pertussis (Tdap) 5
   assessment 52
   bronchitis 55
   catheter site 57
   chickenpox 61
   clostridium difficile-associated diarrhea (CDAD) 60
   control procedures 40–41
   COVID-19 pandemic xi
   diphtheria 5
   gastroenteritis 60
   hepatitis B 7, 23
   hepatitis C virus (HCV) 23
   home care environment and xii
   human immunodeficiency virus/acquired immunodeficiency syndrome (HIV/AIDS) 1, 23
   laboratory-confirmed bloodstream infection (LCBSI) 56–57
   measles, mumps, and rubella (MMR) 5, 61
   N. Meningitis 2
   oral 59
   pertussis (whooping cough) 5, 61
   pneumonia 55
   reinfections xii
   reporting 60–61
   sinusitis 59
   soft tissue 57–58
   symptomatic urinary tract infections (SUTI) 54
   syphilis 23
   tetanus 5
   tuberculosis (TB) 6
influenza-like illness (ILI) 55
IVs in the home environment 39–41

J

John Hopkins Schools of Medicine and Public Health 34

L

laboratory-confirmed bloodstream infection (LCBSI) 56–57

latex gloves 17
legal liability reduction
    discharge summary review 36
    family education 36
    home safety 34
    maintaining patient records 36–38
lower respiratory infections (LRI)
    bronchitis 55
    pneumonia 55
low-risk patient exposure 24

M
MDRO (multidrug-resistant organism) 38
measles, mumps, and rubella (MMR) 61
    acquired immunity 5
    revaccination 5
Medicaid 23
medical records maintenance 36–38
medical waste
    medication disposal 52
    regulations 3
    sharps 3
Medicare 23
MHU (mobile health unit) xii
MIH. *See* mobile-integrated health care (MIH)
MMR. *See* measles, mumps, and rubella (MMR)
mobile health unit (MHU) xii
mobile-integrated health care (MIH) 1
    exposure risks 22
    patient record review 33
    programs 22
multidrug-resistant infections
    EMS communication 38
    patient protocol 38
multidrug-resistant organism (MDRO) 38

N
National Fire Protection Association (NFPA) Standard 1581 6
needle safe devices 16
Needlestick Safety and Prevention Law 16
NFPA (National Fire Protection Association) Standard 1581 6
nitrile gloves 17
N. Meningitis 2

O
Occupational Safety and Health Act of 1970 2
Occupational Safety and Health Administration (OSHA)
    CDC guideline enforcement 6
    General Duty Clause 2, 6–8
    jurisdiction 2–3, 5
OPIM (other potentially infectious materials) 21
oral infections 59
OSHA. *See* Occupational Safety and Health Administration (OSHA)
ostomy care 44–45
other potentially infectious materials (OPIM) 21

P
paramedic scope of practice 22
patients
    care equipment cleaning 31–32
    high-risk 24
    low-risk 24
    maintaining patient records 36–38
    patient record review 33
    testing 23
    understanding 36
PEP Hotline 23
peripherally-inserted central catheters (PICCs) 42
personal protective equipment (PPE)
    CDC guidelines 27
    gloves 17
    home care environment 27–28
    safety controls 15
pertussis (whooping cough) 5, 61
PICCs (peripherally-inserted central catheters) 42
pneumonia 55
postoperative surgical wounds
    caring for 38
    dressing change 38
    EMS training 38
    peripheral site care 40–41
    recording appearance 36
PPE. *See* personal protective equipment (PPE)

precautions 29–30. *See also* contact precautions; transmission-based precautions
   droplet 30
   sharps disposal 49
   standard 29
prehospital emergency care 16, 22
primary bloodstream infection (BSI) 56
Public Health Department 25

R
razor disposal 49, 51
readmission factors 33
reporting 60
   designated infection control officer (DICO) and 23
   infections 60–61
respiratory tract infections and influenza like illness (ILI) 55
Robert Woods Johnson University Hospital 16
Ryan White Comprehensive AIDS Resources Emergency Act
   airborne/droplet exposures 25
   passage 1

S
safety
   checklists 35
   home 34
safety controls 15
   administrative 16
   eliminating 16
   engineering 16
   hierarchy 15
   personal protective equipment (PPE) 16
sharps 3, 16
   contamination 22
   disposal 49
   fingerstick pens disposal 49
   injuries 16
   medical waste 3
   needle safe devices 16
   razor disposal 49, 51
shoes, selection of 48
sinusitis infection 59

skin infections
   fungal 58
   herpes simplex 58
   surgical site infections (SSI) 58
   zoster (shingles) 58
Society for Human Resource Management 7
soft tissue infections 57–58
SOPs (standard operating procedures) 16
specimen transport 52
SSI (surgical site infections) 58
standard operating procedures (SOPs) 16
standard precautions 29
surgical site infections (SSI) 58
symptomatic urinary tract infections (SUTI) 54
syphilis 23

T
TB (tuberculosis) 6
Tdap (acellular pertussis) 5
testing 23
   blood 23–24
tetanus 5
tracheostomy care 45–46
transmission-based precautions
   airborne 30–31
   contact 29–30
   droplet 30
   standard 29
transportation of specimens 52
tuberculosis (TB) 6

U
urinary tract infection (UTI)
   catheter-associated 44, 54
   symptomatic 54

V
vaccines 16
   administration 61
   boosters 5
   costs 5
   declination form 6
   killed-virus 5
   requirements 5–6
   revaccination 5
   Virginia guidelines 61

W

whooping cough (pertussis) 5, 61
work restrictions 7, 13
    COVID-19 pandemic 13
    declination form 6
    employee responsibility 8
    guidelines 7–13
wounds. *See also* postoperative surgical wounds
    irrigation of 51

Z

zoster (shingles) 58